# Bread Machine Cookbook

*Bake Perfect-Every-Time Homemade Bread with Hands-Off Bread Maker Recipes |
Includes Expert Tips, Insiders Secrets & Step-by-Step Instructions*

**Charlize Butt**

# Table of Contents

# Introduction

The familiar, comforting, and nostalgic scent of freshly made bread may take us back in time. It's a smell that makes you think of home and hearth, warm mornings, and sharing a meal with loved ones. Bread has been an essential part of our diets and a symbol of prosperity for millennia.

The idea of making bread from scratch may seem like a pipe dream in today's busy world. Kneading, proofing, and baking the traditional way may be a tedious and time-consuming operation. However, people's craving for the fresh, handcrafted flavor and scent of bread has persisted over the years. Here's where the bread machine shines as an unsung hero of the kitchen, stoking our appetites for handmade treats despite our busy schedules.

Whether you call it a bread machine, bread maker, or something else, it's certain that this incredible equipment has found a permanent home on the counters of homes all over the world. It's a gadget that exemplifies the merging of modern technology with time-honored methods, making it easy for anybody to have access to the delicious benefits of freshly made bread. In this introductory look, we investigate the bread machine, learning about its origins, how it works, and the many options it provides for bakers of all skill levels.

## The Bread Machine: Its Origins and Development

Understanding the bread machine's origins is crucial to fully grasping its significance. Although the idea of using machines to make bread stretches back millennia, the first true bread machine didn't appear until the 1960s.

In the middle of the twentieth century, the concept of a portable bread machine emerged as innovators looked for ways to make baking bread at home easier. The earlier versions were quite simple and relied heavily on human input. More advanced bread machines with automated kneading, rising, and baking cycles were not available until the 1980s, thanks to technological improvements.

Since they became more reasonably priced and simple to operate, bread machines skyrocketed in popularity in the 1990s. These gadgets rapidly became standard in homes all over the world since they were a convenient option for busy families that wanted to enjoy the benefits of baking their own bread. Bread machines have come a long way over the years, with modern models boasting everything from delay timers to adjustable loaf sizes to dedicated gluten-free and artisanal bread programs.

# Explaining How a Bread Maker Operates

A bread machine's primary function is to shorten the time and effort required to bake bread by automating many crucial procedures. A bread machine consists of the bread pan, the kneading paddle or paddles, the control panel, and the heating element. Typically, it goes like this:

- The user measures out flour, liquid (often water or milk), yeast, sugar, salt, and any other optional ingredients like butter, herbs, nuts, or dried fruits before adding them to the bread pan in accordance with the instructions.
- Depending on whether white, whole wheat, French, or sweet bread is required, the user can pick the appropriate program or cycle from the oven's control panel. Some of the more sophisticated machines have functions specifically for preparing dough, jam, and cakes.
- The paddle(s) within the bread machine start to knead and mix the dough. This step is essential for making a cohesive dough and ensuring that all ingredients have been included.
- The machine controls the dough's rising time and temperature. This is where the dough gets its airiness and expands thanks to the carbon dioxide gas produced by the yeast during fermentation.
- Bread machines include a built-in mechanism that switches to the baking phase after the dough has risen. The bread is baked to perfection thanks to the appliance's heating element.
- After baking, most bread machines have a cooling cycle to ensure the bread doesn't become soggy. The newly baked loaf may be removed from the pan when the baking cycle has finished.

The entire procedure is simple and straightforward, so even people with no prior baking knowledge may do it successfully. In what way? A deliciously fragrant loaf of bread on par with those sold at specialty bakeries.

Interestingly, you can make more than just bread in a bread maker. It may be used to make dough for a wide range of foods, from pizza and pasta to cakes. Some versions also include specialized programs for making jams and jellies, expanding the machine's usefulness in the kitchen.

As we explore the bread machine, we learn about its many functions, from making traditional sourdough and hearty multigrain loaves to incorporating unique flavors and textures. This is a trip that honors the merging of modernity and antiquity, turning the age-old process of baking bread into a universally accessible art form.

# Types of Flour Suitable for Bread Machines

### All-Purpose Flour

All-purpose flour is the unsung hero of bread machines, playing a pivotal role in crafting irresistible homemade bread. With its well-balanced protein content, it guarantees the ideal texture for a range of bread varieties. Whether you're whipping up a batch of soft, fluffy white bread or delving into the world of hearty, whole-grain creations, all-purpose flour forms the foundation of your bread machine artistry. It acts as a canvas for your culinary creativity, seamlessly blending with yeast, water, and other ingredients to produce loaves that are a testament to your kitchen prowess. So, in the realm of bread machines, all-purpose flour reigns supreme, ensuring your bread emerges as a delectable masterpiece.

### Bread Flour

Bread flour is the unsung hero in the world of bread machines, elevating your homemade bread to a whole new level of perfection. When it comes to baking in a bread machine, the choice of flour can make all the difference, and bread flour is the star of the show.

What sets bread flour apart is its higher protein content compared to all-purpose flour. This extra protein is essential for developing the gluten structure in your bread, which is crucial for achieving that coveted chewy, yet tender texture in artisanal loaves. When you combine bread flour with yeast, water, and a dash of salt in your bread machine, magic happens.

The bread machine kneads the dough to perfection, and the high-protein content in bread flour ensures that the dough rises beautifully, creating a lofty and airy crumb. The result is bread with a perfect balance of a crisp, golden crust and a soft, chewy interior - just like the ones you'd find in a top-notch bakery.

### Whole Wheat Flour

Whole wheat flour, the unsung hero of healthy baking, takes center stage when it comes to crafting wholesome delights in your trusty bread machine. Its robust, earthy flavor and higher fiber content make it the go-to choice for those seeking nutritious homemade bread.

In the world of bread machines, whole wheat flour introduces a unique twist. It can be a bit trickier to work with compared to all-purpose flour due to its higher protein content, which can result in denser loaves if not handled properly. However, with the right adjustments and a bit of experimentation, you can achieve delightful whole wheat bread that's both nutritious and delicious.

The key lies in finding the perfect balance between whole wheat flour and other ingredients. Many bread machine recipes call for a combination of whole wheat and all-purpose flour to improve the bread's texture and rise. You may also need to increase the liquid content slightly to ensure the dough isn't too dry.

Whole wheat flour offers a range of health benefits, thanks to its whole grain nature. It retains the bran and germ, which are rich in vitamins, minerals, and fiber. This means your homemade bread will not only taste great but also provide essential nutrients for your well-being.

The bread machine simplifies the whole wheat bread-making process, making it accessible to everyone.

## Rye Flour

Rye flour, the often-overlooked sibling of all-purpose flour, brings a unique twist to the world of bread machines. This distinct flour, derived from hearty rye grains, introduces a rich and robust flavor profile to your bread-making endeavors. When integrated into your bread machine recipes, rye flour imparts a delightful earthiness and subtle sweetness, elevating your loaves to a whole new level of taste and complexity.

The magic of rye flour lies in its ability to create dense, hearty bread with a slightly chewy crumb and a characteristically dark crust. It's the secret ingredient behind beloved bread varieties like pumpernickel and traditional European rye bread. And with the convenience of a bread machine, harnessing the potential of rye flour has never been easier.

To make the most of rye flour in your bread machine, it's often combined with all-purpose or bread flour to balance its unique properties. The result? A harmonious blend that captures the best of both worlds – the flavor depth of rye and the structure of wheat flours.

But there's more to rye flour than just taste. It also brings nutritional benefits to the table. Rye is a good source of dietary fiber, vitamins, and minerals, making your homemade bread not only delicious but also nutritious.

## Specialty Flours

Specialty flours bring a unique twist to bread machine baking, elevating your homemade loaves to gourmet status. These specialized flours, such as spelt, rye, or oat flour, offer distinctive flavors and textures that can transform your bread into something truly extraordinary.

When you venture beyond all-purpose flour and experiment with specialty flours, you unlock a world of possibilities. Each type of flour adds its own character to the dough, resulting in bread with nuanced flavors and appealing textures. For instance, spelt flour lends a nutty, slightly sweet taste, while rye flour brings a hearty, earthy note. Oat flour, on the other hand, introduces a subtle sweetness and a tender crumb.

Baking with specialty flours in your bread machine is an adventure in creativity. You can blend different flours to create custom recipes, experimenting with ratios to achieve the perfect balance of flavors and textures. Incorporating these flours also allows you to explore unique bread styles, like rustic European loaves or wholesome multigrain varieties.

Additionally, specialty flours can enhance the nutritional profile of your bread, providing added fiber, vitamins, and minerals. They can be a healthier choice, especially when combined with whole grains.

To make the most of specialty flours in your bread machine, consider recipes specifically designed for these flours or adapt your favorite ones to incorporate them. Keep in mind that some specialty flours may require adjustments to hydration levels or mixing times to achieve optimal results.

# Tricks and Secrets to Bread Machine Mastery

Unlocking the full potential of your bread machine can be a journey filled with delightful surprises. Here, we'll delve into some expert tricks and secrets that will elevate your bread machine mastery to new heights.

Ingredient Precision: Start with high-quality ingredients. Use bread flour for better gluten development and choose fresh yeast or active dry yeast. Pay attention to measurements, especially for liquids, as even slight variations can impact the final result.

**Order of Ingredients**: Always follow the order specified in your bread machine's manual. Typically, liquids go in first, followed by dry ingredients, with yeast added last, often nestled in a small well in the flour to avoid premature activation.

**Yeast Activation:** Proofing the yeast (mixing it with warm water and a pinch of sugar) before adding it to the machine can help ensure its vitality, leading to a better rise and fluffier bread.

**Customization**: Experiment with different flours (whole wheat, rye, or spelt) and various grains (oats, flaxseeds, sunflower seeds) to add depth and texture to your loaves.

**Liquid Adjustment**: Depending on factors like humidity and flour type, you may need to tweak the amount of liquid. Add a tablespoon at a time if the dough appears too dry, or add a bit more flour if it's overly wet.

**Kneading Time**: Let your machine knead the dough for the recommended duration in the manual. Proper kneading is crucial for gluten development and structure.

**Rising Time**: If your machine allows, extend the rising time for a more flavorful bread. Some models have a "rest" or "pause" function that can be used for this purpose.

**Crust Control**: Adjust the crust setting to your preference. For a crispy crust, opt for a darker setting, while a lighter setting will yield a softer crust.

**Add-Ins**: Get creative with add-ins like dried fruits, nuts, or herbs. Add them during the second kneading cycle to ensure even distribution.

**Cooling**: Once your bread is done, resist the urge to slice it immediately. Let it cool on a wire rack for at least 15-20 minutes to avoid a gummy texture.

Cleaning: Clean your bread machine promptly after each use, ensuring that no crumbs or residue remain. This will prolong its lifespan and keep your bread tasting its best.

# Bread Machine Care and Maintenance

Proper care and maintenance of your bread machine are essential for ensuring its longevity and optimal performance. After each use, unplug the machine and allow it to cool. Remove the bread pan, kneading paddle, and other removable parts for cleaning. Wipe down the interior with a damp cloth, being careful not to immerse it in water. Pay attention to the kneading paddle, as residue can accumulate. It's recommended to clean the bread pan and paddle by hand to prevent damage to their non-stick coatings. Regularly check the machine's seals and replace them if they show signs of wear. Following these simple steps will keep your bread machine in top shape, producing delicious loaves for years to come.

### Cleaning Your Machine

Cleaning your bread machine is a crucial yet often overlooked aspect of maintaining its performance and ensuring the longevity of your beloved appliance. While bread machines simplify the bread-making process, they do require regular cleaning to function at their best.

**Start with the basics:** Before anything else, always unplug your bread machine and let it cool down. Remove any breadcrumbs or residual dough from the pan and the kneading paddle. These crumbs can not only affect the flavor of your future loaves but also pose a fire hazard if left unattended.

**The pan and paddle:** Most bread machine pans are non-stick, making them relatively easy to clean. Use warm, soapy water and a gentle sponge to clean the pan and paddle. Avoid using abrasive scrubbers, as they can damage the non-stick coating. If you have stubborn residue, a mixture of baking soda and water can help.

**The exterior:** Wipe down the exterior of your bread machine with a damp cloth to remove any dust or spills. Be cautious not to let any liquid seep into the machine's interior, as it could damage the electrical components.

**The lid and viewing window:** The lid and viewing window can accumulate flour dust and sticky residue over time. Gently clean the lid with a damp cloth, and use a soft, non-abrasive cloth to clean the viewing window. Make sure to dry both thoroughly to prevent moisture from entering the machine.

**Regular maintenance:** In addition to cleaning, consider performing routine maintenance. Check the kneading paddle for signs of wear and tear, and replace it if necessary. Lubricate the machine's moving parts as recommended in the user manual to keep them in optimal condition.

**Deep cleaning:** Periodically, it's a good idea to perform a deep cleaning of your bread machine. Remove the pan, paddle, and other removable parts and wash them thoroughly. Use a can of compressed air to blow out any lingering crumbs or dust from the interior. Always refer to your machine's user manual for specific cleaning instructions.

By taking the time to clean and maintain your bread machine regularly, you'll ensure that it continues to produce delicious, hassle-free loaves for years to come. Proper care not only enhances the machine's performance but also contributes to the overall enjoyment of your homemade bread-making experience.

# Periodic Maintenance

Regular maintenance is crucial for keeping your bread machine in top shape. Here are some essential tips to ensure its longevity:

1. Cleaning: After each use, remove any dough or residue from the baking pan, kneading blade, and interior. Wipe the exterior with a damp cloth.

2. Lubrication: Periodically lubricate moving parts to prevent friction and ensure smooth operation. Consult your user manual for specific instructions.

3. Inspection: Examine the power cord for any damage and check the heating element for signs of wear.

4. Calibration: Test the machine's temperature accuracy by using an oven thermometer during the baking process.

5. Storage: When not in use, store your bread machine in a cool, dry place to prevent moisture buildup.

By following these maintenance steps, you can prolong the life of your bread machine and continue enjoying freshly baked bread.

# Recommended Accessories

When it comes to enhancing your bread machine experience, the right accessories can make a world of difference. Here are some recommended accessories that can elevate your bread-making game.

1. Dough Hook: If your bread machine doesn't come with one, consider getting a dough hook. It simplifies the process of kneading dough, ensuring it's thoroughly mixed and perfectly textured.

2. Bread Pans: Invest in additional bread pans, especially if you plan to experiment with different bread sizes and shapes. Non-stick pans make for easy bread removal.

3. Digital Kitchen Scale: Precision is key in bread making. A digital kitchen scale ensures you measure ingredients accurately, leading to consistent and delicious results.

4. Bread Slicer Guide: Achieve uniform slices with a bread slicer guide. It's a handy tool for those who prefer their bread neatly portioned.

5. Bread Lame: If you're into artisanal bread with decorative slashes, a bread lame is essential. It allows for precise scoring and creates beautiful patterns on the crust.

6. Thermometer: A digital thermometer helps monitor the temperature of your bread's interior. This ensures your bread is perfectly baked and avoids undercooking or overcooking.

7. Silicone Baking Mat: For easy cleanup, consider using silicone baking mats to line your pans. They prevent sticking and make the removal of bread a breeze.

8. Bread Storage Containers: Keep your freshly baked bread fresh longer with airtight storage containers. They maintain the bread's texture and flavor.

9. Ingredient Dispensers: Some bread machines come with ingredient dispensers for adding nuts, seeds, or fruits at the right time during the kneading process. If your machine lacks this feature, you can purchase a separate dispenser.

10. Bread Mixes: For added convenience, try premade bread mixes designed for bread machines. They come in various flavors and styles, making it easy to experiment with different types of bread.

Remember, while these accessories can enhance your bread machine experience, the most crucial element is your passion for creating delicious, homemade bread. Experiment, enjoy the process, and savor the delightful results that your bread machine can deliver with the right tools at your disposal.

Happy baking!

*Chapter 1*

# Basic Breads

## White Bread:

### Ingredients:

- 1 cup of hot (around 110 F/43 C) water
- 2.25 grams of dried active yeast
- Granulated sugar, 2 tablespoons
- About 2 and a half cups of all-purpose flour
- 2 tablespoons of softened unsalted butter
- A pinch and a half of salt

### Instructions:

- Warm the water and add the dried active yeast and sugar to a small bowl. Allow it to rest for 5-10 minutes, or until it begins to foam.
- Flour, butter, and salt should all be placed in the pan of the bread machine. A yeast mixture should be poured in.
- Put the pan into the bread machine and choose the "Basic" or "White Bread" setting. Adjust the crust setting to medium. You may adjust the delay timer on your machine to suit your needs.
- Get the bread maker going, and then relax. It can make dough, let it rise, and bake the bread.
- Carefully remove the bread from the machine once the cycle is complete and set it on a wire rack to cool. Put it in the fridge for half an hour before you try to cut it.

## Brown Bread:

### Ingredients:

- 1 and a quarter cups of room temperature water (around 110 degrees Fahrenheit or 43 degrees Celsius)

- 2.25 grams of dried active yeast
- Molasses, three tablespoons
- 2/3 cup all-purpose flour
- 1/2 a cup of all-purpose flour
- 2 Tablespoons of Oil, Veggie
- A pinch and a half of salt

## Instructions:

- Warm the water and add the dried active yeast and molasses to a small basin. Allow it to rest for 5-10 minutes, or until it begins to foam.
- Put the whole wheat flour, bread flour, vegetable oil, and salt into the pan of the bread machine. A yeast mixture should be poured in.
- Select the "Whole Wheat" or "Brown Bread" setting and insert the pan into the bread maker. Adjust the crust setting to medium. You may adjust the delay timer on your machine to suit your needs.
- Get the bread maker going, and then relax. It can make dough, let it rise, and bake the bread.
- Carefully remove the bread from the machine once the cycle is complete and set it on a wire rack to cool. Wait 30 minutes before cutting into it.

# Chapter 2
# Specialty Breads

## Sourdough Bread:

### Ingredients:

- Starter for sourdough bread, one cup
- 110°F/43°C (about 1 1/2 cups) warm water
- To make bread: 4 cups of flour
- A pinch and a half of salt

### Instructions:

1. Put the sourdough starter, hot water, and bread flour in the pan of the bread machine.
2. Combine the flour and salt.
3. Insert the bread pan and choose the "Sourdough" setting on your bread maker. Adjust the crust setting to medium.
4. Get the bread maker going, and then relax. The sourdough bread will be mixed, let to rise, and baked in it.
5. Carefully remove the bread from the machine once the cycle is complete and set it on a wire rack to cool. Put it in the fridge for half an hour before you try to cut it.

## Multigrain Bread:

### Ingredients:

- 1 and a quarter cups of room temperature water (around 110 degrees Fahrenheit or 43 degrees Celsius)
- 2.25 grams of dried active yeast
- Honey, 3 Tablespoons
- 1/2 a cup of all-purpose flour
- 1 cup of 100% Whole Grain Flour
- Oatmeal, rolled, 1/2 cup

- 1/2 tsp chia seeds
- 1/2 tsp pumpkin seeds
- A pinch and a half of salt

## Instructions:

1. Warm the water, then add the dried yeast and honey to a small basin. Allow it to rest for 5-10 minutes, or until it begins to foam.
2. Mix the bread flour, whole wheat flour, rolled oats, flaxseeds, sunflower seeds, and salt in the bread machine's pan. A yeast mixture should be poured in.
3. Insert the bread pan and choose either the "Whole Wheat" or "Multigrain" setting on your bread maker. Adjust the crust setting to medium.
4. Get the bread maker going, and then relax. The bread maker will mix, knead, and bake the grainy loaf.
5. Carefully remove the bread from the machine once the cycle is complete and set it on a wire rack to cool. Put it in the fridge for half an hour before you try to cut it.

# Gluten-Free Bread:

## Ingredients:

- 110°F/43°C (about 1 1/2 cups) warm water
- 2.25 grams of dried active yeast
- Honey, 3 Tablespoons
- 2 cups all-purpose flour that is gluten-free
- 1/4 pounds ground almonds
- 1/4 cup of ground flaxseed
- Xanthan gum, 1.5 tablespoons
- A pinch and a half of salt

## Instructions:

1. Warm the water, then add the dried yeast and honey to a small basin. Allow it to rest for 5-10 minutes, or until it begins to foam.
2. Put the almond flour, flaxseed meal, xanthan gum, salt, and gluten-free all-purpose flour into the bread machine pan. A yeast mixture should be poured in.
3. Select the "Gluten-Free" cycle and insert the pan into the bread machine. Adjust the crust setting to medium.
4. Get the bread maker going, and then relax. It can prepare gluten-free bread from scratch, from mixing to baking.

5. Carefully remove the bread from the machine once the cycle is complete and set it on a wire rack to cool. Put it in the fridge for half an hour before you try to cut it.

# Vegan Bread:

## Ingredients:

- 1 and a quarter cups of room temperature water (around 110 degrees Fahrenheit or 43 degrees Celsius)
- 2.25 grams of dried active yeast
- Sugar, 3 Tablespoons
- Three Cups of Bread Flour
- 2 Tablespoons of Oil, Veggie
- A pinch and a half of salt

## Instructions:

1. Warm the water and add the dried active yeast and sugar to a small bowl. Allow it to rest for 5-10 minutes, or until it begins to foam.
2. Put the bread flour, oil, and salt into the pan of the bread machine. A yeast mixture should be poured in.
3. Put the pan into the bread machine and choose the "Basic" or "White Bread" setting. Adjust the crust setting to medium.
4. Get the bread maker going, and then relax. Vegan bread will be kneaded, proofed, and baked.
5. Carefully remove the bread from the machine once the cycle is complete and set it on a wire rack to cool. Put it in the fridge for half an hour before you try to cut it.

# Pumpkin bread:

## Ingredients:

- 1 and a quarter cups of room temperature water (around 110 degrees Fahrenheit or 43 degrees Celsius)
- 2.25 grams of dried active yeast
- 3.0 g of dark brown sugar
- 1 cup of chilled, cooked sweet potato mash
- To make bread: 4 cups of flour
- 2 Tablespoons of Oil, Veggie
- A pinch and a half of salt

- An optional 1/2 teaspoon of ground cinnamon.

## Instructions:

1. Warm the water, then add the dried yeast and brown sugar to a small basin. Allow it to rest for 5-10 minutes, or until it begins to foam.
2. To the pan of a bread machine, add the mashed sweet potatoes along with the bread flour, oil, salt, and cinnamon (if using). A yeast mixture should be poured in.
3. Put the pan into the bread machine and choose the "Basic" or "White Bread" setting. Adjust the crust setting to medium.
4. Get the bread maker going, and then relax. The sweet potato bread will be kneaded, risen, and baked.
5. Carefully remove the bread from the machine once the cycle is complete and set it on a wire rack to cool. Wait 30 minutes before cutting into it.

*Chapter 3*

# Spice and Herb Breads

## Rosemary Garlic Bread:

### Ingredients:

- 1 cup of hot (around 110 F/43 C) water
- 2.25 grams of dried active yeast
- Three Cups of Bread Flour
- Granulated sugar, 2 tablespoons
- 4 teaspoons of butter
- A pinch and a half of salt
- Dried Rosemary, 1 Tablespoon
- 2-inches of minced garlic

### Instructions:

1. Warm the water and add the dried active yeast and sugar to a small bowl. Allow it to rest for 5-10 minutes, or until it begins to foam.
2. Pour the yeast mixture, olive oil, salt, dried rosemary, minced garlic, and bread flour into the pan of a bread machine and start the machine.
3. Put your bread maker on the "Basic" or "White Bread" setting. Adjust the crust setting to medium.
4. Get the bread maker going, and then relax. Rosemary garlic bread will be kneaded, risen, and baked.
5. Carefully remove the bread from the machine once the cycle is complete and set it on a wire rack to cool. Put it in the fridge for half an hour before you try to cut it.

## Raisin-Cinnamon Bread:

### Ingredients:

- 1-cup of milk at room temperature (around 43 degrees Celsius/110 degrees Fahrenheit)

- 2.25 grams of dried active yeast
- Three Cups of Bread Flour
- Sugar, Granulated, 1/4 Cup
- 2 tablespoons of softened unsalted butter
- A pinch and a half of salt
- 2 tablespoons of cinnamon powder
- 1 mug of raisins

## Instructions:

1. Warm the milk and stir in the active dry yeast and sugar in a separate small bowl. Allow it to rest for 5-10 minutes, or until it begins to foam.
2. Place the bread flour, butter, salt, cinnamon, raisins, and yeast in the pan of a bread machine.
3. Put your bread maker on the "Basic" or "White Bread" setting. Adjust the crust setting to medium.
4. Get the bread maker going, and then relax. Cinnamon raisin bread will be kneaded, risen, and baked.
5. Carefully remove the bread from the machine once the cycle is complete and set it on a wire rack to cool. Put it in the fridge for half an hour before you try to cut it.

# Herb Bread from Italy:

## Ingredients:

- 1 cup of hot (around 110 F/43 C) water
- 2.25 grams of dried active yeast
- Three Cups of Bread Flour
- 4 teaspoons of butter
- A pinch and a half of salt
- The equivalent of 2 tablespoons of dried oregano, basil, and thyme
- Powdered garlic, 1 teaspoon

## Instructions:

1. Warm the water and add the dried yeast and sugar to a small basin. Allow it to rest for 5-10 minutes, or until it begins to foam.
2. The ingredients for the bread should be placed in the pan of the bread machine: bread flour, olive oil, salt, dried Italian herbs, garlic powder, and the yeast mixture.
3. Put your bread maker on the "Basic" or "White Bread" setting. Adjust the crust setting to medium.

4.  Get the bread maker going, and then relax. Automatically prepares, kneads, rises, and bakes Italian herb bread.
5.  Carefully remove the bread from the machine once the cycle is complete and set it on a wire rack to cool. Put it in the fridge for half an hour before you try to cut it.

# Cheddar and dill bread:

## Ingredients:

- 1 cup of hot (around 110 F/43 C) water
- 2.25 grams of dried active yeast
- Three Cups of Bread Flour
- Sugar, Granulated, 1/4 Cup
- 2 tablespoons of softened unsalted butter
- A pinch and a half of salt
- 2 teaspoons dried dill weed
- Cheddar cheese, one cup's worth

## Instructions:

1.  Warm the water and add the dried active yeast and sugar to a small bowl. Allow it to rest for 5-10 minutes, or until it begins to foam.
2.  Bread flour, butter at room temperature, salt, dried dill, shredded cheddar, and the yeast mixture go into the bread machine pan.
3.  Put your bread maker on the "Basic" or "White Bread" setting. Adjust the crust setting to medium.
4.  Get the bread maker going, and then relax. The machine can make the dough, let it rise, and bake the dill cheddar bread.
5.  Carefully remove the bread from the machine once the cycle is complete and set it on a wire rack to cool. Put it in the fridge for half an hour before you try to cut it.

# Bread with Cheddar and Jalapeños:

## Ingredients:

- 1 cup of hot (around 110 F/43 C) water
- 2.25 grams of dried active yeast
- Three Cups of Bread Flour
- Sugar, Granulated, 1/4 Cup
- 2 tablespoons of softened unsalted butter

- A pinch and a half of salt
- chopped jalapeño peppers, about 1/2 cup (more or less to taste).
- Cheddar cheese, one cup's worth

## Instructions:

1. Warm the water and add the dried active yeast and sugar to a small bowl. Allow it to rest for 5-10 minutes, or until it begins to foam.
2. Bread flour, softened butter, salt, chopped jalapeño peppers, grated cheddar cheese, and the yeast mixture should all go into the bread machine pan.
3. Put your bread maker on the "Basic" or "White Bread" setting. Adjust the crust setting to medium.
4. Get the bread maker going, and then relax. The jalapeño cheddar bread will be kneaded, risen, and baked.
5. Carefully remove the bread from the machine once the cycle is complete and set it on a wire rack to cool. Put it in the fridge for half an hour before you try to cut it.

# Bread with Basil and Sun-Dried Tomatoes:

## Ingredients:

- 1 cup of hot (around 110 F/43 C) water
- 2.25 grams of dried active yeast
- Three Cups of Bread Flour
- Sugar, Granulated, 1/4 Cup
- 4 teaspoons of butter
- A pinch and a half of salt
- 1 cup fresh basil leaves
- Sun-dried tomatoes (in oil) equivalent to 1/2 cup chopped

## Instructions:

1. Warm the water and add the dried active yeast and sugar to a small bowl. Allow it to rest for 5-10 minutes, or until it begins to foam.
2. Put the yeast mixture, olive oil, salt, dried basil, sun-dried tomato chunks, and bread flour in the bread machine pan.
3. Put your bread maker on the "Basic" or "White Bread" setting. Adjust the crust setting to medium.
4. Get the bread maker going, and then relax. The bread will knead, rise, and bake itself with basil and sun-dried tomatoes.

5. Carefully remove the bread from the machine once the cycle is complete and set it on a wire rack to cool. Put it in the fridge for half an hour before you try to cut it.

# Bread with Thyme and Parmesan:

## Ingredients:

- 1 cup of hot (around 110 F/43 C) water
- 2.25 grams of dried active yeast
- Three Cups of Bread Flour
- Sugar, Granulated, 1/4 Cup
- 2 tablespoons of softened unsalted butter
- A pinch and a half of salt
- Dry Thyme, 2 Tablespoons
- Parmesan cheese, grated, 1/2 cup

## Instructions:

1. Warm the water and add the dried active yeast and sugar to a small bowl. Allow it to rest for 5-10 minutes, or until it begins to foam.
2. The ingredients for the bread should be placed in the pan of the bread machine: bread flour, softened butter, salt, dried thyme, grated Parmesan cheese, and the yeast mixture.
3. Put your bread maker on the "Basic" or "White Bread" setting. Adjust the crust setting to medium.
4. Get the bread maker going, and then relax. The bread with thyme and Parmesan will be mixed, let rise, then baked.
5. Carefully remove the bread from the machine once the cycle is complete and set it on a wire rack to cool. Put it in the fridge for half an hour before you try to cut it.

# Onion and Sage Bread:

## Ingredients:

- 1 cup of hot (around 110 F/43 C) water
- 2.25 grams of dried active yeast
- Three Cups of Bread Flour
- Sugar, Granulated, 1/4 Cup
- 2 tablespoons of softened unsalted butter
- A pinch and a half of salt
- Dried sage, 2 teaspoons

- A half cup of chopped onions

## Instructions:

1. Warm the water and add the dried active yeast and sugar to a small bowl. Allow it to rest for 5-10 minutes, or until it begins to foam.
2. Bread flour, butter, salt, dried sage, sliced onions, and yeast mixture should all be placed in the bread machine pan.
3. Put your bread maker on the "Basic" or "White Bread" setting. Adjust the crust setting to medium.
4. Get the bread maker going, and then relax. The sage and onion bread will be kneaded, proofed, and baked.
5. Carefully remove the bread from the machine once the cycle is complete and set it on a wire rack to cool. Put it in the fridge for half an hour before you try to cut it.

# Feta bread with oregano:

## Ingredients:

- 1 cup of hot (around 110 F/43 C) water
- 2.25 grams of dried active yeast
- Three Cups of Bread Flour
- Sugar, Granulated, 1/4 Cup
- 4 teaspoons of butter
- A pinch and a half of salt
- 1 teaspoon of fresh oregano
- a half a cup of feta cheese, crumbled

## Instructions:

1. Warm the water and add the dried active yeast and sugar to a small bowl. Allow it to rest for 5-10 minutes, or until it begins to foam.
2. Mix the yeast with the water and then add the bread flour, olive oil, salt, dried oregano, feta cheese, and the pan from the bread machine.
3. Put your bread maker on the "Basic" or "White Bread" setting. Adjust the crust setting to medium.
4. Get the bread maker going, and then relax. Oregano feta bread will be kneaded, risen, and baked.
5. Carefully remove the bread from the machine once the cycle is complete and set it on a wire rack to cool. Put it in the fridge for half an hour before you try to cut it.

# Bread with Curry Spice:

## Ingredients:

- 1 cup of hot (around 110 F/43 C) water
- 2.25 grams of dried active yeast
- 3 Cups of Bread Flour
- Sugar, Granulated, 1/4 Cup
- 2 tablespoons of softened unsalted butter
- A pinch and a half of salt
- two teaspoons of curry powder

## Instructions:

1. Warm the water and add the dried active yeast and sugar to a small bowl. Allow it to rest for 5-10 minutes, or until it begins to foam.
2. Put the bread flour, butter, salt, curry powder, and yeast in the pan of a bread machine.
3. Put your bread maker on the "Basic" or "White Bread" setting. Adjust the crust setting to medium.
4. Get the bread maker going, and then relax. The bread with curry spices in it will be kneaded, risen, and baked.
5. Carefully remove the bread from the machine once the cycle is complete and set it on a wire rack to cool. Wait 30 minutes before cutting into it.

# Chapter 4

# Seed and Nut Breads

## Sunflower Seed Bread:

### Ingredients:

- 1 cup of hot (around 110 F/43 C) water
- 2.25 grams of dried active yeast
- Three Cups of Bread Flour
- Sugar, Granulated, 1/4 Cup
- 2 tablespoons of softened unsalted butter
- A pinch and a half of salt
- 1/3 mug pumpkin seeds

### Instructions:

1. Warm the water and add the dried active yeast and sugar to a small bowl. Allow it to rest for 5-10 minutes, or until it begins to foam.
2. Put the yeast mixture, sunflower seeds, salt, softened butter, and bread flour in the pan of a bread machine.
3. Put your bread maker on the "Basic" or "White Bread" setting. Adjust the crust setting to medium.
4. Get the bread maker going, and then relax. Sunflower seed bread will be kneaded, risen, and baked.
5. Carefully remove the bread from the machine once the cycle is complete and set it on a wire rack to cool. Put it in the fridge for half an hour before you try to cut it.

## Baking Honey Almond Bread:

### Ingredients:

- 1-cup of milk at room temperature (around 43 degrees Celsius/110 degrees Fahrenheit)
- 2.25 grams of dried active yeast

- Three Cups of Bread Flour
- 1/4 mug of honey
- 2 tablespoons of softened unsalted butter
- A pinch and a half of salt
- Almonds, cut, 1/2 cup

## Instructions:

1. Whisk the dried active yeast, honey, and warm milk together in a small basin. Allow it to rest for 5-10 minutes, or until it begins to foam.
2. Put the yeast mixture, sliced almonds, salt, softened butter, and bread flour in the bread machine pan.
3. Put your bread maker on the "Basic" or "White Bread" setting. Adjust the crust setting to medium.
4. Get the bread maker going, and then relax. Almond honey bread will be kneaded, risen, and baked.
5. Carefully remove the bread from the machine once the cycle is complete and set it on a wire rack to cool. Put it in the fridge for half an hour before you try to cut it.

# Bread with Sesame Seeds:

## Ingredients:

- 1 cup of hot (around 110 F/43 C) water
- 2.25 grams of dried active yeast
- Three Cups of Bread Flour
- Sugar, Granulated, 1/4 Cup
- 2 tablespoons of softened unsalted butter
- A pinch and a half of salt
- 1/2 cup of black sesame seeds

## Instructions:

1. Warm the water and add the dried active yeast and sugar to a small bowl. Allow it to rest for 5-10 minutes, or until it begins to foam.
2. Bread flour, softened butter, salt, sesame seeds, and the yeast mixture go into the bread machine pan.
3. Put your bread maker on the "Basic" or "White Bread" setting. Adjust the crust setting to medium.
4. Get the bread maker going, and then relax. The sesame seed bread will be kneaded, risen, and baked.

5.  Carefully remove the bread from the machine once the cycle is complete and set it on a wire rack to cool. Put it in the fridge for half an hour before you try to cut it.

# Raisin-Walnut Bread:

## Ingredients:

- 1 cup of hot (around 110 F/43 C) water
- 2.25 grams of dried active yeast
- Three Cups of Bread Flour
- Sugar, Granulated, 1/4 Cup
- 2 tablespoons of softened unsalted butter
- A pinch and a half of salt
- 1/4 of an apple diced
- Almonds, 1/2 cup

## Instructions:

1.  Warm the water and add the dried active yeast and sugar to a small bowl. Allow it to rest for 5-10 minutes, or until it begins to foam.
2.  Put the yeast mixture, bread flour, butter that has been melted, salt, chopped walnuts, raisins, and the pan of a bread machine.
3.  Put your bread maker on the "Basic" or "White Bread" setting. Adjust the crust setting to medium.
4.  Get the bread maker going, and then relax. Walnut raisin bread will be kneaded, risen, and baked.
5.  Carefully remove the bread from the machine once the cycle is complete and set it on a wire rack to cool. Put it in the fridge for half an hour before you try to cut it.

# Bread with Flaxseed and Quinoa:

## Ingredients:

- 1 cup of hot (around 110 F/43 C) water
- 2.25 grams of dried active yeast
- Three Cups of Bread Flour
- Sugar, Granulated, 1/4 Cup
- 2 tablespoons of softened unsalted butter
- A pinch and a half of salt
- 1/2 tsp chia seeds

- 1/4 cup of chilled, cooked quinoa

## Instructions:

1. Warm the water and add the dried active yeast and sugar to a small bowl. Allow it to rest for 5-10 minutes, or until it begins to foam.
2. Put the yeast mixture, flaxseeds, cooked and cooled quinoa, and a cup of bread flour in the pan of a bread machine.
3. Put your bread maker on the "Basic" or "White Bread" setting. Adjust the crust setting to medium.
4. Get the bread maker going, and then relax. The flaxseed and quinoa bread will be kneaded, risen, and baked.
5. Carefully remove the bread from the machine once the cycle is complete and set it on a wire rack to cool. Put it in the fridge for half an hour before you try to cut it.

# Bread with Pumpkin Seeds:

## Ingredients:

- 1 cup of hot (around 110 F/43 C) water
- 2.25 grams of dried active yeast
- Three Cups of Bread Flour
- Sugar, Granulated, 1/4 Cup
- 2 tablespoons of softened unsalted butter
- A pinch and a half of salt
- 1/4 cup salted roasted almonds

## Instructions:

1. Warm the water and add the dried active yeast and sugar to a small bowl. Allow it to rest for 5-10 minutes, or until it begins to foam.
2. Put the yeast mixture, roasted pumpkin seeds, salt, melted butter, and bread flour in the pan of a bread machine.
3. Put your bread maker on the "Basic" or "White Bread" setting. Adjust the crust setting to medium.
4. Get the bread maker going, and then relax. The pumpkin seed bread will be kneaded, risen, and baked.
5. Carefully remove the bread from the machine once the cycle is complete and set it on a wire rack to cool. Put it in the fridge for half an hour before you try to cut it.

# Toasty Pecan-Maple Loaf:

## Ingredients:

- 1-cup of milk at room temperature (around 43 degrees Celsius/110 degrees Fahrenheit)
- 2.25 grams of dried active yeast
- Three Cups of Bread Flour
- An Honest Maple Syrup, 14 Cup
- 2 tablespoons of softened unsalted butter
- A pinch and a half of salt
- 1/3 cup finely chopped almonds

## Instructions:

1. Whisk the dried active yeast, maple syrup, and warm milk together in a small basin. Allow it to rest for 5-10 minutes, or until it begins to foam.
2. Bread flour, softened butter, salt, chopped nuts, and the yeast mixture should all go into the bread machine pan.
3. Put your bread maker on the "Basic" or "White Bread" setting. Adjust the crust setting to medium.
4. Get the bread maker going, and then relax. The pecan maple bread will be kneaded, risen, and baked.
5. Carefully remove the bread from the machine once the cycle is complete and set it on a wire rack to cool. Put it in the fridge for half an hour before you try to cut it.

# Jam-Stuffed Buns:

## Ingredients:

- 1 cup of hot (around 110 F/43 C) water
- 2.25 grams of dried active yeast
- Three Cups of Bread Flour
- Sugar, Granulated, 1/4 Cup
- 2 tablespoons of softened unsalted butter
- A pinch and a half of salt
- Poppy seeds, about 2 teaspoons

## Instructions:

1. Warm the water and add the dried active yeast and sugar to a small bowl. Allow it to rest for 5-10 minutes, or until it begins to foam.

2. Bread flour, softened butter, salt, poppy seeds, and yeast mixture should all be placed in the bread machine pan.

3. Put your bread maker on the "Basic" or "White Bread" setting. Adjust the crust setting to medium.

4. Get the bread maker going, and then relax. The poppy seed bread will be kneaded, risen, and baked.

5. Carefully remove the bread from the machine once the cycle is complete and set it on a wire rack to cool. Put it in the fridge for half an hour before you try to cut it.

# Bread with Chia Seeds:

## Ingredients:

- 1 cup of hot (around 110 F/43 C) water
- 2.25 grams of dried active yeast
- Three Cups of Bread Flour
- Sugar, Granulated, 1/4 Cup
- 2 tablespoons of softened unsalted butter
- A pinch and a half of salt
- Use chia seeds, about a quarter cup's worth

## Instructions:

1. Warm the water and add the dried active yeast and sugar to a small bowl. Allow it to rest for 5-10 minutes, or until it begins to foam.

2. Put the yeast mixture, chia seeds, salt, melted butter, and bread flour in the bread machine pan.

3. Put your bread maker on the "Basic" or "White Bread" setting. Adjust the crust setting to medium.

4. Get the bread maker going, and then relax. The bread made with chia seeds will be kneaded, risen, and baked.

5. Carefully remove the bread from the machine once the cycle is complete and set it on a wire rack to cool. Put it in the fridge for half an hour before you try to cut it.

# Baker's Tip for Hazelnut Cranberry Bread:

## Ingredients:

- 1-cup of milk at room temperature (around 43 degrees Celsius/110 degrees Fahrenheit)
- 2.25 grams of dried active yeast

- Three Cups of Bread Flour
- Sugar, Granulated, 1/4 Cup
- 2 tablespoons of softened unsalted butter
- A pinch and a half of salt
- One-half cup of chopped hazelnuts
- Dried Cranberries, 1/2 Cup

## Instructions:

1. Warm the milk and stir in the active dry yeast and sugar in a separate small bowl. Allow it to rest for 5-10 minutes, or until it begins to foam.
2. Place the yeast mixture, bread flour, softened butter, salt, chopped hazelnuts, dried cranberries, and water in the pan of a bread machine and start it.
3. Put your bread maker on the "Basic" or "White Bread" setting. Adjust the crust setting to medium.
4. Get the bread maker going, and then relax. Hazelnut cranberry bread will be kneaded, proofed, and baked.
5. Carefully remove the bread from the machine once the cycle is complete and set it on a wire rack to cool. Wait 30 minutes before cutting into it.

# Chapter 5

# Fruit Breads

## Banana Nut Bread:

### Ingredients:

- Four ripe bananas, mashed to provide one and a half cups.
- 2.25 grams of dried active yeast
- Three Cups of Bread Flour
- Sugar, Granulated, 1/4 Cup
- 2 tablespoons of softened unsalted butter
- A pinch and a half of salt
- 1/4 of an apple diced

### Instructions:

1. Bananas should be mashed and 1 1/2 cups should be measured out.
2. Mix the active dry yeast with the mashed bananas in a small basin. Allow it to rest for 5-10 minutes, or until it begins to foam.
3. Banana yeast mixture, bread flour, granulated sugar, softened butter, salt, chopped walnuts, and a pinch of salt and pepper should all go into the pan of a bread machine.
4. Put your bread maker on the "Basic" or "White Bread" setting. Adjust the crust setting to medium.
5. Get the bread maker going, and then relax. It can mix, raise, and bake a loaf of banana nut bread.
6. Carefully remove the bread from the machine once the cycle is complete and set it on a wire rack to cool. Put it in the fridge for half an hour before you try to cut it.

## Lemon-blueberry bread:

### Ingredients:

- 1 cup of hot (around 110 F/43 C) water
- 2.25 grams of dried active yeast

- Three Cups of Bread Flour
- Sugar, Granulated, 1/4 Cup
- 2 tablespoons of softened unsalted butter
- A pinch and a half of salt
- Lemon gratings one
- 1 cup of blueberries, either fresh or frozen

## Instructions:

1. Warm the water and add the dried active yeast and sugar to a small bowl. Allow it to rest for 5-10 minutes, or until it begins to foam.
2. Place the yeast mixture, fresh or frozen blueberries, lemon zest, salt, and bread flour in the pan of a bread machine.
3. Put your bread maker on the "Basic" or "White Bread" setting. Adjust the crust setting to medium.
4. Get the bread maker going, and then relax. The bread maker will mix, rise, and bake the blueberry lemon bread.
5. Carefully remove the bread from the machine once the cycle is complete and set it on a wire rack to cool. Put it in the fridge for half an hour before you try to cut it.

# Orange and cranberry bread:

## Ingredients:

- 1 cup of hot (around 110 F/43 C) water
- 2.25 grams of dried active yeast
- Three Cups of Bread Flour
- Sugar, Granulated, 1/4 Cup
- 2 tablespoons of softened unsalted butter
- A pinch and a half of salt
- The rind of one orange
- Dried cranberries, one cup

## Instructions:

1. Warm the water and add the dried active yeast and sugar to a small bowl. Allow it to rest for 5-10 minutes, or until it begins to foam.
2. Place the bread flour, butter, salt, orange zest, dried cranberries, and yeast mixture in the pan of a bread machine and start the machine.
3. Put your bread maker on the "Basic" or "White Bread" setting. Adjust the crust setting to medium.

4. Get the bread maker going, and then relax. The cranberry orange bread will be kneaded, risen, and baked.

5. Carefully remove the bread from the machine once the cycle is complete and set it on a wire rack to cool. Put it in the fridge for half an hour before you try to cut it.

# Cinnamon and apple bread:

## Ingredients:

- 1 cup of hot (around 110 F/43 C) water
- 2.25 grams of dried active yeast
- Three Cups of Bread Flour
- Sugar, Granulated, 1/4 Cup
- 2 tablespoons of softened unsalted butter
- A pinch and a half of salt
- Apples (such as Granny Smiths): 2 cups, peeled, cored, and cut
- 1 tsp of cinnamon powder

## Instructions:

1. Warm the water and add the dried active yeast and sugar to a small bowl. Allow it to rest for 5-10 minutes, or until it begins to foam.

2. Flour, butter, salt, apples, cinnamon, and yeast should all go into the bread machine pan.

3. Put your bread maker on the "Basic" or "White Bread" setting. Adjust the crust setting to medium.

4. Get the bread maker going, and then relax. Apple cinnamon bread will be kneaded, risen, and baked.

5. Carefully remove the bread from the machine once the cycle is complete and set it on a wire rack to cool. Put it in the fridge for half an hour before you try to cut it.

# Almond-cherry bread:

## Ingredients:

- 1 cup of hot (around 110 F/43 C) water
- 2.25 grams of dried active yeast
- Three Cups of Bread Flour
- Sugar, Granulated, 1/4 Cup
- 2 tablespoons of softened unsalted butter
- A pinch and a half of salt

- Dried Cherries, One Cup
- 1/4 pound of sliced almonds

## Instructions:

1. Warm the water and add the dried active yeast and sugar to a small bowl. Allow it to rest for 5-10 minutes, or until it begins to foam.
2. Place the bread flour, butter, salt, dried cherries, almonds, and yeast in the pan of a bread machine and start the machine.
3. Put your bread maker on the "Basic" or "White Bread" setting. Adjust the crust setting to medium.
4. Get the bread maker going, and then relax. Cherry almond bread will be kneaded, risen, and baked.
5. Carefully remove the bread from the machine once the cycle is complete and set it on a wire rack to cool. Put it in the fridge for half an hour before you try to cut it.

# Bread with Figs and Walnuts:

## Ingredients:

- 1 cup of hot (around 110 F/43 C) water
- 2.25 grams of dried active yeast
- Three Cups of Bread Flour
- Sugar, Granulated, 1/4 Cup
- 2 tablespoons of softened unsalted butter
- A pinch and a half of salt
- 1 cup of dried figs, chopped
- 1/4 of an apple diced

## Instructions:

1. Warm the water and add the dried active yeast and sugar to a small bowl. Allow it to rest for 5-10 minutes, or until it begins to foam.
2. Put the yeast mixture, chopped dried figs, chopped walnuts, and the yeast in the bread machine pan.
3. Put your bread maker on the "Basic" or "White Bread" setting. Adjust the crust setting to medium.
4. Get the bread maker going, and then relax. It can make dough, let it rise, and bake a loaf of fig and walnut bread.
5. Carefully remove the bread from the machine once the cycle is complete and set it on a wire rack to cool. Put it in the fridge for half an hour before you try to cut it.

# Ginger bread with peaches:

## Ingredients:

- 1 cup of hot (around 110 F/43 C) water
- 2.25 grams of dried active yeast
- Three Cups of Bread Flour
- Sugar, Granulated, 1/4 Cup
- 2 tablespoons of softened unsalted butter
- A pinch and a half of salt
- 1 cup of peaches, either fresh or canned, chopped
- Crystallized ginger, minced, 2 teaspoons

## Instructions:

1. Warm the water and add the dried active yeast and sugar to a small bowl. Allow it to rest for 5-10 minutes, or until it begins to foam.
2. Place the yeast mixture, bread flour, butter, salt, peaches, crystallized ginger, and minced ginger in the pan of a bread machine.
3. Put your bread maker on the "Basic" or "White Bread" setting. Adjust the crust setting to medium.
4. Get the bread maker going, and then relax. The peach ginger bread will be mixed, raised, and baked.
5. Carefully remove the bread from the machine once the cycle is complete and set it on a wire rack to cool. Put it in the fridge for half an hour before you try to cut it.

# Coconut and pineapple bread:

## Ingredients:

- 1 cup of hot (around 110 F/43 C) water
- 2.25 grams of dried active yeast
- Three Cups of Bread Flour
- Sugar, Granulated, 1/4 Cup
- 2 tablespoons of softened unsalted butter
- A pinch and a half of salt
- One-half cup of crushed, drained pineapple
- One-half cup of coconut flakes

## Instructions:

1. Warm the water and add the dried active yeast and sugar to a small bowl. Allow it to rest for 5-10 minutes, or until it begins to foam.
2. Flour, butter, salt, crushed pineapple, coconut, and yeast should all go into the bread machine pan.
3. Put your bread maker on the "Basic" or "White Bread" setting. Adjust the crust setting to medium.
4. Get the bread maker going, and then relax. Pineapple coconut bread will be kneaded, risen, and baked.
5. Carefully remove the bread from the machine once the cycle is complete and set it on a wire rack to cool. Put it in the fridge for half an hour before you try to cut it.

# Chapter 6
# Vegetable Breads

## Zucchini Parmesan Bread:

Ingredients:

- Shredded zucchini (with extra liquid squeezed out): 1 1/2 cups
- 2.25 grams of dried active yeast
- Three Cups of Bread Flour
- Parmesan cheese, grated, 1/4 cup
- 2 tablespoons of softened unsalted butter
- A pinch and a half of salt
- Powdered garlic, half a teaspoon

Instructions:

1. Shred the zucchini and use a clean dish towel or paper towels to wring out any excess liquid.
2. Shred the zucchini and put it in a small dish with the active dry yeast. Allow it to rest for 5-10 minutes, or until it begins to foam.
3. Put the zucchini yeast mixture, bread flour, grated Parmesan cheese, softened butter, salt, garlic powder, and baking powder into the bread machine's pan.
4. Put your bread maker on the "Basic" or "White Bread" setting. Adjust the crust setting to medium.
5. Get the bread maker going, and then relax. The bread maker will make the dough for the zucchini Parmesan bread and bake it when it has risen.
6. Carefully remove the bread from the machine once the cycle is complete and set it on a wire rack to cool. Put it in the fridge for half an hour before you try to cut it.

## Raisin and carrot bread:

Ingredients:

- carrots, shredded, 1 1/2 cups
- 14 cup dried fruit

- 2.25 grams of dried active yeast
- Three Cups of Bread Flour
- Add 2 tbsp. of honey
- 2 tablespoons of softened unsalted butter
- A pinch and a half of salt
- 1/4 of a teaspoon of cinnamon powder

## Instructions:

1. The carrots should be grated and kept aside.
2. Grate the carrots and place them in a small dish together with the raisins and active dry yeast. Allow it to rest for 5-10 minutes, or until it begins to foam.
3. Spread the yeast mixture, carrot raisin combination, honey, softened butter, salt, ground cinnamon, and bread flour in the pan of a bread machine.
4. Put your bread maker on the "Basic" or "White Bread" setting. Adjust the crust setting to medium.
5. Get the bread maker going, and then relax. Carrot and raisin bread will be kneaded, proofed, and baked.
6. Carefully remove the bread from the machine once the cycle is complete and set it on a wire rack to cool. Put it in the fridge for half an hour before you try to cut it.

# Pan Bread with Spinach and Feta:

## Ingredients:

- 1 cup of chopped, wilted fresh spinach
- a half a cup of feta cheese, crumbled
- 2.25 grams of dried active yeast
- Three Cups of Bread Flour
- 4 teaspoons of butter
- A pinch and a half of salt
- Dry Oregano, 1/2 Teaspoon

## Instructions:

1. Fresh spinach should be chopped and rapidly sautéed to wilt it. The temperature needs to drop a bit.
2. Melt the butter and add the active dry yeast to the wilted spinach in a small dish. Allow it to rest for 5-10 minutes, or until it begins to foam.
3. Put the bread flour, olive oil, salt, dried oregano, and the yeast mixture made from the spinach and feta in the bread machine's pan.

4. Put your bread maker on the "Basic" or "White Bread" setting. Adjust the crust setting to medium.

5. Get the bread maker going, and then relax. Spinach and feta bread will be kneaded, risen, and baked.

6. Carefully remove the bread from the machine once the cycle is complete and set it on a wire rack to cool. Put it in the fridge for half an hour before you try to cut it.

# Bread with Sweet Potatoes and Pecans:

## Ingredients:

- 1 cup of chilled, cooked sweet potato mash
- 1/3 cup finely chopped almonds
- 2.25 grams of dried active yeast
- Three Cups of Bread Flour
- Add 2 tbsp. of honey.
- 2 tablespoons of softened unsalted butter
- A pinch and a half of salt
- 1/4 of a teaspoon of cinnamon powder

## Instructions:

1. The sweet potatoes should be cooked, mashed, and allowed to cool.

2. Mash the sweet potatoes and add the active dry yeast and chopped pecans to a small bowl. Allow it to rest for 5-10 minutes, or until it begins to foam.

3. Put the sweet potato pecan yeast mixture, honey, melted butter, salt, ground cinnamon, and bread flour in the bread machine pan.

4. Put your bread maker on the "Basic" or "White Bread" setting. Adjust the crust setting to medium.

5. Get the bread maker going, and then relax. The sweet potato and pecan bread will be kneaded, risen, and baked.

6. Carefully remove the bread from the machine once the cycle is complete and set it on a wire rack to cool. Put it in the fridge for half an hour before you try to cut it.

# Baking using Butternut Squash:

## Ingredients:

- 1 cup of cooked, mashed butternut squash.
- 2.25 grams of dried active yeast

- Three Cups of Bread Flour
- Add 2 tbsp. of honey.
- 2 tablespoons of softened unsalted butter
- A pinch and a half of salt
- Nutmeg, ground, 1/2 teaspoon

## Instructions:

1. Prepare the butternut squash by cooking it and mashing it.
2. Mash the butternut squash and add the active dry yeast to a small basin. Allow it to rest for 5-10 minutes, or until it begins to foam.
3. Throw the yeast mixture for the butternut squash into the bread machine along with the bread flour, honey, softened butter, salt, and grated nutmeg.
4. Put your bread maker on the "Basic" or "White Bread" setting. Adjust the crust setting to medium.
5. Get the bread maker going, and then relax. Butternut squash bread will be kneaded, risen, and baked.
6. Carefully remove the bread from the machine once the cycle is complete and set it on a wire rack to cool. Put it in the fridge for half an hour before you try to cut it.

# Baking Bread with Onions and Chives:

## Ingredients:

- One-half cup of cooked and cooled onion chunks
- Chopped fresh chives, 2 teaspoons
- 2.25 grams of dried active yeast
- Three Cups of Bread Flour
- 2 tablespoons of softened unsalted butter
- A pinch and a half of salt
- Onion powder equaling 1/2 teaspoon

## Instructions:

1. Prepare the translucent onion by chopping and sautéing it. Just give them some time to calm off.
2. Cooked onions, fresh chives, and active dry yeast should be combined in a small basin. Allow it to rest for 5-10 minutes, or until it begins to foam.
3. Bread flour, softened butter, salt, onion powder, and onion chive yeast combination should all be placed in the bread machine pan.

4. Put your bread maker on the "Basic" or "White Bread" setting. Adjust the crust setting to medium.
5. Get the bread maker going, and then relax. To make onion and chive bread, it will knead, let the dough rise, and bake it.
6. Carefully remove the bread from the machine once the cycle is complete and set it on a wire rack to cool. Put it in the fridge for half an hour before you try to cut it.

# Bread with Beets and Goat Cheese:

## Ingredients:

- Cooked and cooled beets, half a cup grated
- Goat cheese, crumbled, 1/2 cup
- 2.25 grams of dried active yeast
- Three Cups of Bread Flour
- 4 teaspoons of butter
- A pinch and a half of salt
- One-fourth of a teaspoon of pepper

## Instructions:

1. Grate the beets once they have cooled.
2. Grated beets, crumbled goat cheese, and active dry yeast should be mixed together in a small basin. Allow it to rest for 5-10 minutes, or until it begins to foam.
3. Bread flour, olive oil, salt, black pepper, and the beet goat cheese yeast combination put into the bread machine pan.
4. Put your bread maker on the "Basic" or "White Bread" setting. Adjust the crust setting to medium.
5. Get the bread maker going, and then relax. The bread will knead, rise, and bake with the addition of the beets and goat cheese.
6. Carefully remove the bread from the machine once the cycle is complete and set it on a wire rack to cool. Put it in the fridge for half an hour before you try to cut it.

# Cheddar bread with broccoli:

## Ingredients:

- Cooked and cooled broccoli florets (about 1/2 cup)
- 1/4 of a block of cream cheese
- 2.25 grams of dried active yeast

- Three Cups of Bread Flour
- 2 tablespoons of softened unsalted butter
- A pinch and a half of salt
- A Garlic Powder Measurement Equal to One-Fourth of a Tablespoon

## Instructions:

1. Once the broccoli florets have cooled, chop them.
2. Add the cheddar cheese, active dry yeast, and broccoli to a small bowl and mix well. Allow it to rest for 5-10 minutes, or until it begins to foam.
3. Broccoli cheddar yeast mixture, bread flour, melted butter, salt, garlic powder, and bread machine pan.
4. Put your bread maker on the "Basic" or "White Bread" setting. Adjust the crust setting to medium.
5. Get the bread maker going, and then relax. The broccoli cheddar bread will be kneaded, risen, and baked.
6. Carefully remove the bread from the machine once the cycle is complete and set it on a wire rack to cool. Put it in the fridge for half an hour before you try to cut it.

# Bread with Roasted Red Peppers:

## Ingredients:

- Chopped roasted red peppers equaling 1/2 cup
- 2.25 grams of dried active yeast
- Three Cups of Bread Flour
- 4 teaspoons of butter
- A pinch and a half of salt
- One-half of a teaspoon of basil powder

## Instructions:

1. Roasted red peppers should be chopped.
2. Mix the active dry yeast with the chopped roasted red peppers in a small dish. Allow it to rest for 5-10 minutes, or until it begins to foam.
3. To the pan of a bread machine, add bread flour, olive oil, salt, dried basil, and the yeast combination from the roasted red peppers.
4. Put your bread maker on the "Basic" or "White Bread" setting. Adjust the crust setting to medium.
5. Get the bread maker going, and then relax. The roasted red pepper bread will be mixed, proofed, and baked.

6. Carefully remove the bread from the machine once the cycle is complete and set it on a wire rack to cool. Put it in the fridge for half an hour before you try to cut it.

# Garlic bread and kale:

## Ingredients:

- 1 cup of cooked, cooled kale, chopped
- 2-inches of minced garlic
- 2.25 grams of dried active yeast
- Three Cups of Bread Flour
- 4 teaspoons of butter
- A pinch and a half of salt
- One-half teaspoon of dried thyme

## Instructions:

1. When the kale is done cooking, cut it up.
2. Stir the garlic powder, active dry yeast, and chopped kale together in a small basin. Allow it to rest for 5-10 minutes, or until it begins to foam.
3. Put the kale garlic yeast combination, the kale, and the bread flour in the bread machine pan.
4. Put your bread maker on the "Basic" or "White Bread" setting. Adjust the crust setting to medium.
5. Get the bread maker going, and then relax. Automatically mix, raise, and bake a loaf of kale and garlic bread.
6. Carefully remove the bread from the machine once the cycle is complete and set it on a wire rack to cool. Wait 30 minutes before cutting into it.

*Chapter 7*
# Gluten-free Breads

## Gluten-Free White Bread:

### Ingredients:

- Gluten-free all-purpose flour, about 1 1/2 cups
- Xanthan gum, 1.5 tablespoons
- 2.25 grams of dried active yeast
- One and a half teaspoons of white sugar
- A pinch and a half of salt
- 1 and a quarter cups of room temperature water (around 110 degrees Fahrenheit or 43 degrees Celsius)
- Veggie Oil, a Quarter Cup
- Three huge eggs

### Instructions:

1. Warm water, sugar, and dried active yeast should be mixed in a separate basin. Allow it to rest for 5-10 minutes, or until it begins to foam.
2. Put the gluten-free all-purpose flour, xanthan gum, salt, oil, and eggs into the bread machine pan.
3. The yeast mixture should be poured into the pan.
4. If your bread machine has a setting for it, use the "Gluten-Free" setting. In any other case, select the medium crust option on the "Basic" or "White Bread" cycle.
5. Get the bread maker going, and then relax. To make gluten-free white bread, it will knead, raise, and bake the dough.
6. Carefully remove the bread from the machine once the cycle is complete and set it on a wire rack to cool. Put it in the fridge for half an hour before you try to cut it.

# Grain-free, gluten-free bread:

## Ingredients:

- 1 1/2 cups of whole-grain gluten-free flour
- Xanthan gum, 1.5 tablespoons
- 2.25 grams of dried active yeast
- Half a cup of honey
- A pinch and a half of salt
- 1 and a quarter cups of room temperature water (around 110 degrees Fahrenheit or 43 degrees Celsius)
- Veggie Oil, a Quarter Cup
- Three huge eggs

## Instructions:

1. Mix honey, active dry yeast, and warm water in a small basin. Allow it to rest for 5-10 minutes, or until it begins to foam.
2. Gluten-free whole grain flour mix, xanthan gum, salt, vegetable oil, and eggs should all be placed in the bread machine pan.
3. The yeast mixture should be poured into the pan.
4. If your bread machine has a setting for it, use the "Gluten-Free" setting. In any other case, select the medium crust option on the "Basic" or "White Bread" cycle.
5. Get the bread maker going, and then relax. To make gluten-free whole grain bread, it will knead, raise, and bake the ingredients.
6. Carefully remove the bread from the machine once the cycle is complete and set it on a wire rack to cool. Put it in the fridge for half an hour before you try to cut it.

# Banana Bread without Gluten:

## Ingredients:

- Gluten-free all-purpose flour, about 1 1/2 cups
- Xanthan gum, 1.5 tablespoons
- 2.25 grams of dried active yeast
- A pinch and a half of salt
- Veggie Oil, a Quarter Cup
- Sugar, Granulated, 1/4 Cup
- The mashed flesh of 2 very ripe bananas

- 1/2 cup of apple sauce, unsweetened
- Exactly one vanilla extract teaspoon

## Instructions:

1. Mix active dry yeast with mashed bananas in a small basin. Allow it to rest for 5-10 minutes, or until it begins to foam.
2. Put the gluten-free all-purpose flour, xanthan gum, salt, oil, sugar, applesauce, and vanilla extract into the bread machine's pan.
3. The banana yeast mixture should be poured into the pan.
4. If your bread machine has a setting for it, use the "Gluten-Free" setting. In any other case, select the medium crust option on the "Basic" or "White Bread" cycle.
5. Get the bread maker going, and then relax. The gluten-free banana bread will be kneaded, risen, and baked.
6. Carefully remove the bread from the machine once the cycle is complete and set it on a wire rack to cool. Put it in the fridge for half an hour before you try to cut it.

# Seed and nut bread that is free of gluten:

## Ingredients:

- Gluten-free all-purpose flour, about 1 1/2 cups
- Xanthan gum, 1.5 tablespoons
- 2.25 grams of dried active yeast
- A pinch and a half of salt
- Veggie Oil, a Quarter Cup
- almonds, walnuts, or another type of chopped nut, 1/4 cup
- 2 tablespoons of a variety of seeds (such as flax, chia, and sunflower)
- 1 and a quarter cups of room temperature water (around 110 degrees Fahrenheit or 43 degrees Celsius)

## Instructions:

1. Warm water and dried active yeast should be mixed in a small basin. Allow it to rest for 5-10 minutes, or until it begins to foam.
2. Put the yeast mixture, xanthan gum, salt, vegetable oil, nuts, seeds, and gluten-free all-purpose flour in the bread machine pan and turn it on.
3. If your bread machine has a setting for it, use the "Gluten-Free" setting. In any other case, select the medium crust option on the "Basic" or "White Bread" cycle.
4. Get the bread maker going, and then relax. Gluten-free seed and nut bread will be kneaded, risen, and baked.

5. Carefully remove the bread from the machine once the cycle is complete and set it on a wire rack to cool. Put it in the fridge for half an hour before you try to cut it.

# Blueberry Bread that is Free of Gluten:

## Ingredients:

- Gluten-free all-purpose flour, about 1 1/2 cups
- Xanthan gum, 1.5 tablespoons
- 2.25 grams of dried active yeast
- A pinch and a half of salt
- Veggie Oil, a Quarter Cup
- Sugar, Granulated, 1/4 Cup
- 1 1/2 cups of blueberries, either fresh or frozen
- Exactly one vanilla extract teaspoon

## Instructions:

1. Mix active dry yeast with blueberries, either fresh or frozen, in a small basin. Allow it to rest for 5-10 minutes, or until it begins to foam.
2. Put the gluten-free all-purpose flour, xanthan gum, salt, oil, sugar, and vanilla extract into the bread machine's pan.
3. Blueberry yeast mixture should be added to the pan.
4. If your bread machine has a setting for it, use the "Gluten-Free" setting. In any other case, select the medium crust option on the "Basic" or "White Bread" cycle.
5. Get the bread maker going, and then relax. To make gluten-free blueberry bread, it will knead, raise, and bake the dough.
6. Carefully remove the bread from the machine once the cycle is complete and set it on a wire rack to cool. Put it in the fridge for half an hour before you try to cut it.

# Cinnamon raisin bread gluten:

## Ingredients:

- Gluten-free all-purpose flour, about 1 1/2 cups
- Xanthan gum, 1.5 tablespoons
- 2.25 grams of dried active yeast
- A pinch and a half of salt
- Veggie Oil, a Quarter Cup
- Sugar, Granulated, 1/4 Cup

- One and a half tablespoons of cinnamon powder
- Almonds, 1/2 cup
- 1 and a quarter cups of room temperature water (around 110 degrees Fahrenheit or 43 degrees Celsius)

## Instructions:

1. Warm water, sugar, ground cinnamon, and active dry yeast should be mixed in a small basin. Allow it to rest for 5-10 minutes, or until it begins to foam.
2. Put the yeast mixture, xanthan gum, salt, vegetable oil, raisins, and gluten-free all-purpose flour in the bread machine pan.
3. If your bread machine has a setting for it, use the "Gluten-Free" setting. In any other case, select the medium crust option on the "Basic" or "White Bread" cycle.
4. Get the bread maker going, and then relax. Gluten-free cinnamon raisin bread will be kneaded, risen, and baked.
5. Carefully remove the bread from the machine once the cycle is complete and set it on a wire rack to cool. Put it in the fridge for half an hour before you try to cut it.

# Pumpkin Bread:

## Ingredients:

- Gluten-free all-purpose flour, about 1 1/2 cups
- Xanthan gum, 1.5 tablespoons
- 2.25 grams of dried active yeast
- A pinch and a half of salt
- Veggie Oil, a Quarter Cup
- Sugar, Granulated, 1/4 Cup
- Half a cup of pumpkin puree from a can
- The Pumpkin Spice Mixture, 1 Teaspoon
- 1 and a quarter cups of room temperature water (around 110 degrees Fahrenheit or 43 degrees Celsius)

## Instructions:

1. Put the pumpkin puree, pumpkin spice, and active dry yeast into a small basin and mix well. Allow it to rest for 5-10 minutes, or until it begins to foam.
2. Gluten-free all-purpose flour, xanthan gum, salt, vegetable oil, granulated sugar, and the yeast mixture should all be placed in the bread machine pan.
3. If your bread machine has a setting for it, use the "Gluten-Free" setting. In any other case, select the medium crust option on the "Basic" or "White Bread" cycle.

4. Get the bread maker going, and then relax. The gluten-free pumpkin bread will be kneaded, risen, and baked.

5. Carefully remove the bread from the machine once the cycle is complete and set it on a wire rack to cool. Put it in the fridge for half an hour before you try to cut it.

# Quinoa bread without gluten:

## Ingredients:

- Gluten-free all-purpose flour, about 1 1/2 cups
- Xanthan gum, 1.5 tablespoons
- 2.25 grams of dried active yeast
- A pinch and a half of salt
- Veggie Oil, a Quarter Cup
- 1/4 cup cooled cooked quinoa
- 1 and a quarter cups of room temperature water (around 110 degrees Fahrenheit or 43 degrees Celsius)

## Instructions:

1. Once the quinoa has cooled, mix in the active dry yeast in a small dish. Allow it to rest for 5-10 minutes, or until it begins to foam.

2. Put the yeast mixture, xanthan gum, salt, vegetable oil, and gluten-free all-purpose flour in the bread machine's pan.

3. If your bread machine has a setting for it, use the "Gluten-Free" setting. In any other case, select the medium crust option on the "Basic" or "White Bread" cycle.

4. Get the bread maker going, and then relax. The machine will make the dough, let the quinoa bread rise, and bake the loaf.

5. Carefully remove the bread from the machine once the cycle is complete and set it on a wire rack to cool. Put it in the fridge for half an hour before you try to cut it.

# Yeast-Free Bread with Sunflower Seeds:

## Ingredients:

- Gluten-free all-purpose flour, about 1 1/2 cups
- Xanthan gum, 1.5 tablespoons
- 2.25 grams of dried active yeast
- A pinch and a half of salt
- Veggie Oil, a Quarter Cup

- 1/2 tsp pumpkin seeds
- 1 and a quarter cups of room temperature water (around 110 degrees Fahrenheit or 43 degrees Celsius)

## Instructions:

1. Combine active dry yeast and sunflower seeds in a small basin. Allow it to rest for 5-10 minutes, or until it begins to foam.
2. Put the yeast mixture, xanthan gum, salt, vegetable oil, and gluten-free all-purpose flour in the bread machine's pan.
3. If your bread machine has a setting for it, use the "Gluten-Free" setting. In any other case, select the medium crust option on the "Basic" or "White Bread" cycle.
4. Get the bread maker going, and then relax. Sunflower seed bread that is devoid of gluten will be kneaded, fermented, and baked.
5. Carefully remove the bread from the machine once the cycle is complete and set it on a wire rack to cool. Put it in the fridge for half an hour before you try to cut it.

# Chocolate Chip Bread without Gluten:

## Ingredients:

- Gluten-free all-purpose flour, about 1 1/2 cups
- Xanthan gum, 1.5 tablespoons
- 2.25 grams of dried active yeast
- A pinch and a half of salt
- Veggie Oil, a Quarter Cup
- 1/2 a jar of peanut butter
- 1 and a quarter cups of room temperature water (around 110 degrees Fahrenheit or 43 degrees Celsius)

## Instructions:

1. Mix the active dry yeast and chocolate chips in a small dish. Allow it to rest for 5-10 minutes, or until it begins to foam.
2. Put the yeast mixture, xanthan gum, salt, vegetable oil, and gluten-free all-purpose flour in the bread machine's pan.
3. If your bread machine has a setting for it, use the "Gluten-Free" setting. In any other case, select the medium crust option on the "Basic" or "White Bread" cycle.
4. Get the bread maker going, and then relax. It will mix, raise, and bake the bread with gluten-free chocolate chips.

5. Carefully remove the bread from the machine once the cycle is complete and set it on a wire rack to cool. Wait 30 minutes before cutting into it.

*Chapter 8*
# Cheese Breads

## Cheddar and Jalapeño Bread:

### Ingredients:

- Cheese, shredded cheddar: 1 1/2 cups
- Seeded and thinly sliced jalapeo peppers (1-2)
- 2.25 grams of dried active yeast
- Three Cups of Bread Flour
- 2 tablespoons of softened unsalted butter
- A pinch and a half of salt
- Powdered garlic, 1 teaspoon

### Instructions:

1. Shredded cheddar cheese, chopped jalapeos, and active dry yeast should all be mixed together in a small basin. Allow it to rest for 5-10 minutes, or until it begins to foam.
2. Bread flour, unsalted butter, salt, garlic powder, and the cheese-jalapeo yeast combination should all be placed in the bread machine pan.
3. Put your bread maker on the "Basic" or "White Bread" setting. Adjust the crust setting to medium.
4. Get the bread maker going, and then relax. To make cheddar and jalapeo bread, it will knead, rise, and bake the dough.
5. Carefully remove the bread from the machine once the cycle is complete and set it on a wire rack to cool. Put it in the fridge for half an hour before you try to cut it.

## Garlic Bread with Parmesan:

### Ingredients:

- 1 cup of freshly grated Parmesan
- 3 minced garlic cloves

- 2.25 grams of dried active yeast
- Three Cups of Bread Flour
- 2 tablespoons of softened unsalted butter
- A pinch and a half of salt
- Dry Oregano, 1/2 Teaspoon

## Instructions:

1. Mix the minced garlic, active dry yeast, and grated Parmesan cheese in a small basin. Allow it to rest for 5-10 minutes, or until it begins to foam.
2. Bread flour, unsalted butter, salt, dried oregano, and the Parmesan garlic yeast combination should all be placed in the bread machine pan.
3. Put your bread maker on the "Basic" or "White Bread" setting. Adjust the crust setting to medium.
4. Get the bread maker going, and then relax. Parmesan garlic bread will be kneaded, risen, and baked.
5. Carefully remove the bread from the machine once the cycle is complete and set it on a wire rack to cool. Put it in the fridge for half an hour before you try to cut it.

# Bread with Gouda and Onions:

## Ingredients:

- One and a half cups of shredded Gouda
- Onions, 1/2 cup, chopped finely
- 2.25 grams of dried active yeast
- Three Cups of Bread Flour
- 2 tablespoons of softened unsalted butter
- A pinch and a half of salt
- One-half teaspoon of dried thyme

## Instructions:

1. Shred the Gouda cheese and add it to a small dish with the chopped onions and active dry yeast. Allow it to rest for 5-10 minutes, or until it begins to foam.
2. Bread flour, unsalted butter, salt, dried thyme, and the Gouda onion yeast combination should all be placed in the bread machine pan.
3. Put your bread maker on the "Basic" or "White Bread" setting. Adjust the crust setting to medium.
4. Get the bread maker going, and then relax. The Gouda and onion bread will be kneaded, risen, and baked.

5. Carefully remove the bread from the machine once the cycle is complete and set it on a wire rack to cool. Put it in the fridge for half an hour before you try to cut it.

# Bread with Asiago and Rosemary:

## Ingredients:

- 1 1/2 cups of Asiago cheese, shredded
- Chopped fresh rosemary equal to 1 tablespoon
- 2.25 grams of dried active yeast
- Three Cups of Bread Flour
- 2 tablespoons of softened unsalted butter
- A pinch and a half of salt
- Powdered garlic, half a teaspoon

## Instructions:

1. Shred some Asiago cheese and mix it with some fresh rosemary and active dry yeast in a small basin. Allow it to rest for 5-10 minutes, or until it begins to foam.
2. Put the ingredients for the bread in the pan of a bread machine: bread flour, unsalted butter, salt, garlic powder, and the yeast combination made from Asiago and rosemary.
3. Put your bread maker on the "Basic" or "White Bread" setting. Adjust the crust setting to medium.
4. Get the bread maker going, and then relax. The bread with Asiago and rosemary in it will be kneaded, risen, and baked.
5. Carefully remove the bread from the machine once the cycle is complete and set it on a wire rack to cool. Put it in the fridge for half an hour before you try to cut it.

# Bread with Brie and Cranberries:

## Ingredients:

- 1 1/2 ounces of cubed Brie
- Dried Cranberries, 1/2 Cup
- 2.25 grams of dried active yeast
- Three Cups of Bread Flour
- 2 tablespoons of softened unsalted butter
- A pinch and a half of salt
- 1/4 mug of honey

**Instructions:**

1. Cube the Brie and blend it with the dried cranberries and active dry yeast in a small dish. Allow it to rest for 5-10 minutes, or until it begins to foam.
2. Throw in the ingredients for the bread in the pan of your bread machine: bread flour, unsalted butter, salt, honey, and the yeast, cranberry, and Brie combination.
3. Put your bread maker on the "Basic" or "White Bread" setting. Adjust the crust setting to medium.
4. Get the bread maker going, and then relax. Brie and cranberry bread will be mixed, proofed, and baked.
5. Carefully remove the bread from the machine once the cycle is complete and set it on a wire rack to cool. Put it in the fridge for half an hour before you try to cut it.

# Bread with Blue Cheese and Walnuts:

**Ingredients:**

- Blue cheese, crumbled, about 1 1/2 cups
- 1/4 of an apple diced
- 2.25 grams of dried active yeast
- Three Cups of Bread Flour
- 2 tablespoons of softened unsalted butter
- A pinch and a half of salt
- One-fourth of a teaspoon of pepper

**Instructions:**

1. Crumble the blue cheese, cut the walnuts, and add the active dry yeast to a small basin. Allow it to rest for 5-10 minutes, or until it begins to foam.
2. Place the bread flour, unsalted butter, salt, pepper, and blue cheese walnut yeast mixture in the pan of a bread machine and turn it on.
3. Put your bread maker on the "Basic" or "White Bread" setting. Adjust the crust setting to medium.
4. Get the bread maker going, and then relax. The bread with blue cheese and walnuts will be mixed, risen, and baked in the machine.
5. Carefully remove the bread from the machine once the cycle is complete and set it on a wire rack to cool. Put it in the fridge for half an hour before you try to cut it.

# Bread with Tomatoes and Mozzarella:

## Ingredients:

- 1 1/2 cups of mozzerella cheese, shredded
- One-half cup of chopped tomatoes (canned, drained).
- 2.25 grams of dried active yeast
- Three Cups of Bread Flour
- 2 tablespoons of softened unsalted butter
- A pinch and a half of salt
- 1/2 fresh basil leaf

## Instructions:

1. Shredded mozzarella cheese, chopped tomatoes, and active dry yeast should be mixed together in a small basin. Leave it alone for 5-10 minutes to foam up.
2. Bread flour, unsalted butter, salt, dried basil, and the mozzarella tomato yeast combination should all be placed in the bread machine pan.
3. Put your bread maker on the "Basic" or "White Bread" setting. Adjust the crust setting to medium.
4. Turn on the bread maker and walk away. The bread with mozzarella and tomatoes in it will be kneaded, risen, and baked.
5. Carefully remove the bread from the machine once the cycle is complete and set it on a wire rack to cool. Don't cut into it for at least half an hour after it's finished cooling.

# Bagel with Gruyère and Bacon:

## Ingredients:

- Gruyère cheese, shredded, about 1 1/2 cups
- Half a cup of bacon, cooked and crumbled
- 2.25 grams of dried active yeast
- Three Cups of Bread Flour
- 2 tablespoons of softened unsalted butter
- A pinch and a half of salt
- One-half teaspoon of dried thyme

## Instructions:

1. Shred the Gruyère cheese and add it to the dish with the crumbled bacon and active dry yeast. Leave it alone for 5-10 minutes to foam up.

2. Put the yeast mixture for the Gruyère bacon, bread flour, unsalted butter, salt, dried thyme, and bread in the bread machine's pan.
3. Put your bread maker on the "Basic" or "White Bread" setting. Adjust the crust setting to medium.
4. Turn on the bread maker and walk away. The Gruyère and bacon bread will be kneaded, fermented, and baked.
5. Carefully remove the bread from the machine once the cycle is complete and set it on a wire rack to cool. Wait 30 minutes before cutting into it.

*Chapter 9*

# Sweet Breads

## Cinnamon Raisin Bread:

### Ingredients:

- 1 cup of hot (around 110 F/43 C) water
- 2.25 grams of dried active yeast
- Three cups of bread flour
- 2 tbsp. of white sugar
- 2 tablespoons of softened unsalted butter
- A pinch and a half of salt
- One and a half tablespoons of cinnamon powder
- 1 mug of raisins

### Instructions:

1. Warm the water and add the dried active yeast and sugar to a small bowl. Leave it alone for 5-10 minutes to foam up.
2. Put the bread flour, the melted butter, the salt, and the cinnamon in the pan of your bread machine. Put in the yeast and sugar.
3. Put your bread maker on the "Basic" or "White Bread" setting. Adjust the crust setting to medium.
4. Turn on the bread maker and walk away. Cinnamon raisin bread will be kneaded, risen, and baked.
5. Add the raisins to the dough about 10 minutes before the end of the kneading process.
6. Carefully remove the bread from the machine once the cycle is complete and set it on a wire rack to cool. Don't cut into it for at least half an hour after it's finished cooling.

## Banana Nut Bread:

### Ingredients:

- 1-cup of milk at room temperature (around 43 degrees Celsius/110 degrees Fahrenheit)

- 2.25 grams of dried active yeast
- Three cups of bread flour
- Sugar, Granulated, 1/4 Cup
- 2 tablespoons of softened unsalted butter
- A pinch and a half of salt
- 1/4 cup chopped nuts

### Instructions:

1. Warm the milk and stir in the active dry yeast and sugar in a separate small bowl. Leave it alone for 5-10 minutes to foam up.
2. Put the chocolate chips, salt, softened butter, and bread flour in the pan of a bread machine. Put in the yeast and sugar.
3. Put your bread maker on the "Basic" or "White Bread" setting. Adjust the crust setting to medium.
4. Turn on the bread maker and walk away. The bread maker will mix, raise, and bake the chocolate chip bread.
5. Carefully remove the bread from the machine once the cycle is complete and set it on a wire rack to cool. Don't cut into it for at least half an hour after it's finished cooling.

# Sliced Banana Bread:

### Ingredients:

- The mashed flesh of 2 very ripe bananas
- 1/4 cup of hot (around 110 F/43 C) water
- 2.25 grams of dried active yeast
- Three cups of bread flour
- Sugar, Granulated, 1/4 Cup
- 2 tablespoons of softened unsalted butter
- A pinch and a half of salt
- Walnuts, chopped (optional) 1/2 cup

### Instructions:

1. Warm the water and add the dried active yeast and sugar to a small bowl. Leave it alone for 5-10 minutes to foam up.
2. Put the mashed bananas, bread flour, softened butter, salt, and (optionally) chopped walnuts into the pan of your bread machine. Put in the yeast and sugar.
3. Put your bread maker on the "Basic" or "White Bread" setting. Adjust the crust setting to medium.

4. Turn on the bread maker and walk away. It can mix, raise, and bake a loaf of banana bread for you.

5. Carefully remove the bread from the machine once the cycle is complete and set it on a wire rack to cool. Don't cut into it for at least half an hour after it's finished cooling.

# Blueberry and lemon bread:

## Ingredients:

- 1 cup of hot (around 110 F/43 C) water
- 2.25 grams of dried active yeast
- Three cups of bread flour
- Sugar, Granulated, 1/4 Cup
- 2 tablespoons of softened unsalted butter
- A pinch and a half of salt
- Lemon gratings one
- 1 cup of blueberries, either fresh or frozen

## Instructions:

1. Warm the water and add the dried active yeast and sugar to a small bowl. Leave it alone for 5-10 minutes to foam up.

2. Throw in some blueberries, some lemon zest, some salt, some melted butter, and some bread flour into the pan of your bread machine. Put in the yeast and sugar.

3. Put your bread maker on the "Basic" or "White Bread" setting. Adjust the crust setting to medium.

4. Turn on the bread maker and walk away. Lemon blueberry bread will be kneaded, risen, and baked.

5. Carefully remove the bread from the machine once the cycle is complete and set it on a wire rack to cool. Wait 30 minutes before cutting into it.

# Chapter 10
# Holiday and Festive Breads

## Easter Bread:

### Ingredients:

- Milk, half a cup, warmed at around 110 degrees Fahrenheit (43 degrees Celsius).
- 2 Dry yeast, active: one-fourth teaspoon
- Sugar, Granulated, 1/4 Cup
- 1/2 cup of softened unsalted butter
- Four big eggs
- 4 cups all-purpose flour
- 1/2 milligram of salt
- Vanilla extract, half a teaspoon
- 1/2 cup of candied fruit mixture (citrus, cherry, etc.)
- Almonds, chopped (optional) 1/4 cup

### Instructions:

1. Warm the milk and stir in the active dry yeast and sugar in a separate small bowl. Leave it alone for 5-10 minutes to foam up.
2. Put the cubed butter, eggs, bread flour, salt, and vanilla essence in the pan of a bread machine. Put in the yeast and sugar.
3. Turn on your bread machine and choose the "Dough" or "Manual" setting. The dough will rise and be kneaded throughout this cycle, but it won't be baked.
4. At the end of the dough cycle, take the dough out of the machine and lay it on a floured work surface. Mix in the optional candied fruit and nuts with a little kneading.
5. Form the dough into an Easter bread form, such as a braid.
6. Bread should rise for 1 hour, or until doubled in size, on a greased baking sheet covered with a clean kitchen towel.
7. Start by setting the oven temperature to 175 degrees Celsius (or 350 degrees Fahrenheit). Make sure the Easter bread is golden brown and hollow when you tap the bottom of the pan. This should take around 25 to 30 minutes.
8. Bread should be served after cooling on a wire rack.

# Christmas Stollen:

## Ingredients:

- Milk, half a cup, warmed at around 110 degrees Fahrenheit (43 degrees Celsius).
- 2.25 grams of dried active yeast
- Sugar, Granulated, 1/4 Cup
- 1/2 cup of softened unsalted butter
- Size of 2 big eggs
- 3 and a half cups bread flour
- 1/2 milligram of salt
- Chopped candied fruits (such as citron or cherries) equals 1/2 cup.
- 1/4 pound of sliced almonds
- Almonds, 1/2 cup
- 1 tsp of cinnamon powder
- Nutmeg, ground, one-fourth teaspoon
- Dusting sugar from the bakery

## Instructions:

1. Warm the milk and stir in the active dry yeast and sugar in a separate small bowl. Leave it alone for 5-10 minutes to foam up.
2. Softened butter, eggs, bread flour, salt, cinnamon, nutmeg, and the yeast mixture should all be placed in the bread machine pan. Turn on your bread machine and choose the "Dough" or "Manual" setting.
3. At the end of the dough cycle, take the dough out of the machine and lay it on a floured work surface. Mix in the dried fruit, nuts, and raisins by kneading them in.
4. Roll the dough out into an oval or a log.
5. Let the formed dough rest for an hour, or until doubled in size, on a baking sheet coated with cooking spray.
6. Start by setting the oven temperature to 175 degrees Celsius (or 350 degrees Fahrenheit). If you want a golden brown Stollen, bake it for 30-35 minutes.
7. The Stollen should be let to cool for a few minutes before being liberally dusted with confectioners' sugar.

# Christmas Bread:

## Ingredients:

- 1 cup of hot (around 110 F/43 C) water

- 2.25 grams of dried active yeast
- Sugar, Granulated, 1/4 Cup
- Veggie Oil, a Quarter Cup
- Three huge eggs
- 4 cups all-purpose flour
- A pinch and a half of salt
- Toppings of poppy or sesame seeds (both optional).

## Instructions:

1. Warm the water and add the dried active yeast and sugar to a small bowl. Leave it alone for 5-10 minutes to foam up.
2. Put the yeast mixture, salt, sugar, vegetable oil, bread flour, and eggs in the bread machine pan. Turn on your bread machine and choose the "Dough" or "Manual" setting.
3. At the end of the dough cycle, take the dough out of the machine and lay it on a floured work surface.
4. Cut the dough in half, then in half again. To make a challah, roll each piece into a rope and then braid them together.
5. The challah should be let to rise for 30-45 minutes, or until somewhat puffy, on a greased baking sheet covered with a clean kitchen towel.
6. Start by setting the oven temperature to 175 degrees Celsius (or 350 degrees Fahrenheit). The challah can be brushed with an egg wash and sprinkled with poppy or sesame seeds if desired.
7. To test if the challah is done, tap the bottom of the pan; it should sound hollow.
8. Before serving, let the challah cool on a wire rack.

# Cornbread with Thanksgiving:

## Ingredients:

- One Cup of Cornmeal
- 1/4 cup self-rising flour
- Sugar, Granulated, 1/4 Cup
- Baking powder, one tablespoon
- 1/2 milligram of salt
- Size of 2 big eggs
- 1 glass milk
- a melted 1/4 cup of unsalted butter
- Veggie Oil, a Quarter Cup

## Instructions:

1. Mix the cornmeal, all-purpose flour, sugar, baking powder, and salt together in a large basin.
2. Eggs, milk, melted butter, and vegetable oil should all be mixed together in a separate basin after being beaten. Blend together effectively.
3. Combine the wet and dry components by pouring the wet into the dry and stirring together.
4. Cornbread batter should be transferred to the pan of a bread machine.
5. Activate the bread machine's "Bake-Only" or "Cake" setting. If you like a thinner crust, choose the medium setting.
6. Get the cornbread baking in the bread machine. The oven will take care of baking.
7. Carefully remove the cornbread from the machine once the cycle is complete, and allow it to cool for a few minutes before slicing and serving.

*Chapter 11*

# Troubleshooting and FAQs

## Common Issues and How to Solve Them

Although bread makers make it easy to have freshly baked bread at home, they are nonetheless subject to the same wear and tear as any other kitchen item. If you're serious about creating bread, you should know how to fix these common issues. The most common problems with bread makers and their fixes are discussed here.

### Trouble with Dry or Wet Dough:

Getting the dough to the appropriate consistency is one of the most prevalent challenges. Add water, one teaspoon at a time, until the dough comes together into a smooth ball, if necessary. If the dough is too sticky and moist, add flour, one teaspoon at a time, until the desired consistency is reached.

### Baking Without Success:

Make sure your yeast is fresh if your bread isn't rising. Yeast that's been sitting around for too long won't rise. Too hot or too cold liquid might influence yeast activity, so make sure your liquid components are at the proper temperature, usually around 110°F (43C). Also, check that the yeast quantity you're using is appropriate for the recipe.

### Bread Sinks or Collapses:

It's possible that your bread lost its structure because it rose too much during baking. Over-fermentation can be avoided by lowering the yeast concentration or cutting back on the sugar content.

### Too Much Bread Weighs You Down:

Too much mixing of the dough or not allowing it to rise enough might cause a dense or heavy loaf. Make sure the dough has doubled in size during the rising period and mix and knead for the timeframes specified in your bread machine's user manual. A heavy loaf might also be the consequence of using too much flour, so be careful when measuring.

## Bad Smell or Taste in the Bread:

The quality of your ingredients or the water you used might be to blame if your bread has an undesirable flavor or odor. Check the expiration dates on all of your components, but especially the flour and yeast. If the tap water in your area has an unpleasant smell or flavor, you may want to switch to a different water source.

## The Crust of Bread Is White:

If the bread machine isn't set to bake at a high enough temperature or for long enough, the crust will be too pale. Make sure the bread machine is set to the proper cycle for the bread you intend to bake. You may control the degree of browning of the crust on some models.

## Fried Breadsticks:

Make sure you grease the bread pan well with butter, oil, or nonstick cooking spray so your bread doesn't cling. It may be simpler to remove the loaf from the pan if you line the bottom with parchment paper.

## Too Much Booming or Shaking:

whether your bread machine is making strange noises or vibrating excessively, check to see whether the paddle is striking the sides of the pan. Make sure the paddle is secured securely and the machine is sitting on a flat, solid surface.

## Trouble with the Bread Maker:

When the cycle of your bread maker abruptly ends, the motor may have overheated. Let it cool down for a while before you try to restart the machine. If the problem remains, it's probably an electrical one, and you should call the manufacturer.

## Inconsistent Browning or Raising:

If the ingredients aren't spread out equally in the bread pan, the bread may rise unevenly or bake unevenly. When placing the dough in the pan, be careful to do it evenly. To achieve even mixing, stop the machine periodically throughout the blending process and scrape down the edges.

## Fault Detection and Repair:

Some more sophisticated bread machines will display an error code if there is a problem. Check your machine's handbook for solutions if you get an error message. If a problem persists, you should get in touch with the manufacturer.

## Strange Odors or Smoke:

Turn off and disconnect your bread maker immediately if you smell something strange or see smoke emanating from it. These symptoms may point to an underlying mechanical or electrical issue that needs to be checked out. Please wait for the machine to be examined before attempting to use it.

While bread machines might make certain steps easier, they are not foolproof. Sticking to the recipe as written, using only fresh ingredients, and keeping the machine in good working order should fix most issues. Keeping the paddles and the pan clean and clear of residue on a regular basis also helps avoid problems. Check your bread machine's handbook or get in touch with customer service if you run across any issues that don't seem to be resolved. Delicious handmade bread may be created in a bread machine with some skill and troubleshooting.

# Frequently Asked Questions

### 1. What is a bread machine, and how does it work?

A bread machine, often called a bread maker, is a device used to create bread through an automated process. A bread machine has a pan, paddles for kneading the dough, a control panel, and a heating source. Simply said, you load the bread pan with materials (flour, water, yeast, etc.), choose a program, and let the machine handle the rest, including mixing, kneading, rising, and baking. The baking process relies on the heat generated by the heating element.

### 2. Besides making bread, what else can I create in a bread machine?

Though they are usually used for baking bread, bread machines may also be used to make other types of dough (pizza, pasta, etc.) and even some types of cake. Jam and gluten-free bread options are available on certain more sophisticated versions.

### 3. What are the must-haves while using a bread machine to bake bread?

To make bread with a bread machine, you'll need flour, water, yeast, sugar, salt, and a fat source (like oil or butter). Milk, eggs, herbs, spices, and nuts are just a few examples of what may be added to alter the flavor.

### 4. Can I use all-purpose flour for bread flour?

Most bread machine recipes will work OK with all-purpose flour in place of bread flour. Bread flour, on the other hand, has more protein, which can improve the bread's texture and rise. If you're using all-purpose flour instead, you might need to increase the amount slightly to get the same texture.

### 5. When making bread in a bread machine, how much of each component should I use?

Accurate ingredient measurement is essential. Flour and other dry components require dry measuring cups, whereas liquids like water and milk require liquid measuring cups. Use a flat edge to level off dry ingredients, and measure liquids at eye level, for the most accurate results.

## 6. When making bread in a bread machine, can I use either active dry yeast or quick yeast?

Bread machines can utilize either active dry yeast or quick yeast. Because it doesn't require proving in water before being added to dry ingredients, instant yeast is favored by many. Before adding active dried yeast to the bread machine, it should be proofed in warm water with a pinch of sugar.

## 7. If I want to keep my yeast for a long time, what should I do?

Keep your yeast frozen in an airtight container. Yeast, if preserved correctly, may maintain its viability for a year or longer.

## 8. Can I use a bread machine to create gluten-free bread?

Gluten-free bread may be made in a bread machine. Make gluten-free bread by following a mix's instructions or a recipe developed specifically for your bread maker. If you've ever made ordinary bread in your machine before, you'll want to make sure it's completely clean.

## 9. There was a problem with the rise of my bread. Where may the problem lie?

Bread rising can be influenced by a number of factors:

- The yeast you use must be active and not over its expiration date.
- Yeast activation occurs at a water temperature of around 110 degrees Fahrenheit (43 degrees Celsius).
- Measurement errors: Correct component amounts are critical.
- Make sure the machine kneads the dough well throughout the kneading cycle.

Recipes may need to be adapted at high altitudes.

## 10. If my bread turns out too dense, what can I do?

Overmixing or inadequate rise might cause a thick loaf. Take a look at this:

- Ensure the dough is kneaded for the correct amount of time in the machine.
- Allow the dough to rise until it has doubled in size.
- Too much flour can make the bread dense, so be careful when measuring it out.

## 13. When I bake bread, it always seems to stick to the pan.

In order to avoid sticking:

- Butter, oil, or nonstick cooking spray the bread pan.
- To make cleaning the pan a breeze, line it with parchment paper.

## 12. Why does my bread's crust look so white?

If the bread machine isn't set to bake at a high enough temperature or for long enough, the crust will be too pale. If your bread machine has a crust setting, use it, otherwise look for a new recipe.

## 13. Can I alter the bread by adding things like nuts, seeds, or dried fruits?

Nuts, seeds, dried fruits, and even chocolate chips can be added to bread to enhance its flavor and texture. During the kneading or mixing portion of your machine's cycle is when you should add these ingredients.

## 14. When was the last time you cleaned your bread machine?

A machine's lifespan can be significantly increased with regular cleaning and servicing. After each usage, make sure you unplug the bread maker and take out the bread pan and kneading paddles. These components should be cleaned with warm, soapy water and then dried completely. Apply a moist towel to the inside of the machine and wipe it down. For further information on how to clean your device, go to the handbook.

## 15. If an error code appears on the screen of my bread maker, how can I fix it?

Specific problems are indicated by error codes. For a complete rundown of possible malfunctions and how to fix them, consult the machine's user guide. If the issue persists, get in touch with the manufacturer.

## 16. Can I use a conventional bread maker to create gluten-free bread?

Although you may use a conventional bread maker to bake gluten-free bread, a machine designed for the purpose is preferred. The special requirements of gluten-free bread are more easily met by these machines because of the specific settings they often provide.

## 17. I live at a high altitude, yet none of my baking recipes work.

Baking is impacted by the reduced air pressure seen at higher elevations. Recipe modifications may involve:

- Lessen the amount of yeast.
- Boost your fluid intake (milk/water).
- Modify the baking duration and heat.
- Find the optimal ratio for your altitude by experimenting.

## 18. When I bake sourdough bread, can I use a bread machine?

Although bread machines aren't perfect for sourdough fermentation, they may be used to make bread that tastes similar to sourdough. Use the dough option to mix and knead the dough according to a sourdough bread recipe. Then, prior to baking, the dough is given the usual sourdough fermentation treatment.

### 19. The question is whether or not whole wheat flour can be used in a bread maker.

Whole wheat flour may be used in a bread maker. Denser bread may be the outcome of using whole wheat flour. For enhanced texture and rise, try using a mix of whole wheat and bread flour.

### 20. Can I trust the bread machine and walk away while it bakes?

Once the baking cycle has begun, you can usually leave the bread maker alone. However, if you're trying a new recipe, it's best to stick around for the first combining and kneading stages.

*Bonus Chapter*

# Beyond Bread

## Making Jam in Your Bread Machine:

Ingredients:

- 4 cups of fruit, either fresh or frozen (blueberries, raspberries, peaches, etc.).
- 1 1/2 cups of white sugar, granulated
- Lemon juice, 1 tablespoon
- 1 tablespoon of pectin (for extra thickness, if desired).

Instructions:

1. Prepare the fruit by washing it. Larger fruits, such as peaches, should be chopped up before using.
2. Fill the pan of your bread machine with the fruit, sugar, lemon juice, and pectin (if using).
3. The "Jam" or "Jam Setting" must be chosen on the bread machine. Use the "Quick" setting if your machine doesn't have a jam setting.
4. Get the jam cooking in the machine and get it going. Count on spending between 60 and 90 minutes on this.
5. Jam consistency should be checked periodically. Add additional pectin and keep heating if it's not thickening enough.
6. Once the jam has thickened to your liking, remove the pan from the mixer and set it aside to cool. As it cools, it will thicken even more.
7. Refrigerate the jam after you've transferred it to sanitized jars.

# Using a Bread Machine to Prepare Pizza Dough:

Ingredients:

- 1 cup of hot (around 110 F/43 C) water
- 2.25 grams of dried active yeast
- 2 and a half cups bread flour
- 1 tsp. sugar

- 1.25 grams of salt
- 4 teaspoons of butter

## Instructions:

1. Warm the water and add the dried active yeast and sugar to a small bowl. Leave it alone for 5-10 minutes to foam up.
2. Put the bread flour, salt, and olive oil into the pan of the bread machine. Put in the yeast and sugar.
3. Turn on your bread machine and choose the "Dough" or "Manual" setting.
4. At the end of the dough cycle, take the dough out of the machine and lay it on a floured work surface.
5. Flatten the dough into a pizza of the appropriate size and thickness.
6. Place the dough on a pizza stone or parchment-lined baking sheet.
7. Put in a preheated oven at 475 degrees Fahrenheit (245 degrees Celsius) for 12 to 15 minutes, or until the crust is toasted and the cheese is bubbling and browned.

# Using a Bread Machine to Make Pasta Dough:

## Ingredients:

- 4 cups bread flour
- Size of 2 big eggs
- A Cup and a Half of Water
- 1/2 milligram of salt

## Instructions:

1. All-purpose flour and salt should be placed in the pan of the bread maker.
2. Beat the egg with the water in a separate bowl.
3. Add the egg mixture to the flour in the pan of the bread maker and start the machine.
4. Turn on your bread machine and choose the "Dough" or "Manual" setting.
5. At the end of the dough cycle, take the dough out of the machine and lay it on a floured work surface.
6. Make the spaghetti as thin or as thick as you choose by rolling out the dough. A pasta maker or rolling pin will do the trick here.
7. Make fettuccine, spaghetti, or lasagna sheets, or any other pasta shape you choose.
8. Fresh pasta needs only a few minutes in boiling salted water to reach the perfect al dente texture. The pasta's thickness determines how long it needs to cook.
9. Put the cooked pasta on a plate and top it with whatever you choose.

# Conclusion

It's safe to say that the bread machine changed how we bake at home forever. The convenience of having freshly made bread on hand without the time-consuming effort of baking it by hand has led to the widespread adoption of this multifunctional device. Several major findings and observations emerge when we consider our time spent in the bread machine universe.

First and foremost, the bread machine allows people with varying degrees of baking experience to experience the satisfaction of making their own bread. The bread machine is useful whether you're a seasoned baker looking for a time-saving method to create artisan loaves or a complete baking newbie. Its user-friendly layout and pre-set options streamline the process while guaranteeing reliably tasty results every time. This has inspired many others to try their hand at baking bread and experimenting in the kitchen.

The bread machine's adaptability is one of its most appealing features. It works with not only the more common white or whole wheat loaves, but also sourdough, multigrain, gluten-free, and fruit breads. Home bakers may now personalize their bread to their own tastes and dietary restrictions by experimenting with a wide range of ingredients, flavors, and textures in their own kitchens.

In addition, the bread machine has encouraged culinary innovation and creativity. Those with a passion for baking have expanded into the world of artisanal bread, creating unique varieties flavored with herbs, spices, cheeses, fruits, and nuts. The options are practically endless, inspiring chefs to experiment with their baking skills and skills in the kitchen.

The bread machine is a lifesaver for people who are always on the go because of how much time it saves. Time is valuable, and being able to make bread or dough with minimum effort saves a lot of it. With freshly made bread waiting to be toasted or converted into sandwiches, even the busiest mornings become more doable. The ease and pleasure the bread machine gives to daily life are evidenced by the scent of freshly made bread drifting through the kitchen.

While the bread machine's convenience cannot be denied, it is nevertheless a tool that keeps the basics of bread-making intact. It maintains the time-honored practice of using just flour, water, yeast, and salt in its breads. Because it incorporates cutting-edge tools with time-tested methods, it serves as a link between the past and the present.

The bread machine has shown its practical and financial benefits. People who bake their own bread at home may choose the highest quality ingredients and avoid buying processed bread from the grocery store. This has a multiplicative effect on the health benefits gained and the money saved over time.

Along the way, we've covered the most frequent problems with bread makers and how to fix them. We've covered the ins and outs of using a bread machine, from getting the dough to rise just so to deciphering problem messages. If you're serious about baking, you need to know these problems and how to fix them.

In conclusion, the bread machine is now a standard appliance in many households. It has leveled the playing field when it comes to baking bread, making it possible for everyone to make their own loaves. It has revitalized home baking and sparked a newfound appreciation for cooking as a result of its adaptability, portability, and creative potential. The timeless pleasure of sharing a meal with loved ones is commemorated with each bite of warm, homemade bread as we toast the perfect balance between history and modernity, taste and utility. Our lives have been improved by the bread machine in more ways than one.

Made in the USA
Columbia, SC
28 December 2023

29598140R00046